THE KNOWLEDGE

THE POWER OF

menopause & midlife

BY DR NIGHAT ARIF

hamlyn

hamlyn

First published as *The Power of Menopause & Midlife*
in Great Britain in 2025 by Hamlyn, an imprint of
Octopus Publishing Group Ltd
Carmelite House
50 Victoria Embankment
London EC4Y 0DZ
www.octopusbooks.co.uk

An Hachette UK Company
www.hachette.co.uk

The authorized representative in the EEA is Hachette Ireland,
8 Castlecourt Centre, Dublin 15, D15 XTP3, Ireland (email: info@hbgi.ie)

This material was previously published as *The Knowledge: Your guide to female health from menstruation to the menopause* by Aster in 2023

ISBN 978-0-60063-974-9
eISBN 978-0-60063-975-6

A CIP catalogue record for this book is available from the British Library.

Typeset in 10.5/15pt Sabon LT Pro by Six Red Marbles UK, Thetford, Norfolk

Printed and bound in Great Britain.

1 3 5 7 9 10 8 6 4 2

This FSC® label means that materials used for the product have been responsibly sourced.

FSC www.fsc.org MIX Paper | Supporting responsible forestry FSC® C104740

Disclaimer: Before making any changes in your health regime, or starting any medical treatment, always consult your own doctor for advice relevant to your individual circumstances.

Staff Credits:
Publisher: Kate Fox
Senior Editor: Pauline Bache
Art Director: Jaz Bahra
Words Contributor: Joanne Lake
Illustrator: Liliana Rasmussen
Picture Research: Giulia Hetherington and Jennifer Veall
Copy Editor: Joanne Smith
Production Manager: Caroline Alberti

THE POWER OF

menopause & midlife

CONTENTS

YOUR GUIDE TO FEMALE HEALTH

Back in the spring of 2019, I was working at a practice in rural Buckinghamshire as a GP with a special interest in women's health. That area of medicine had always fascinated me, from menstruation through to menopause, and helping people to access the right care and treatment had become my vocation and my passion.

Alongside my GP duties, I began to create social media posts to raise awareness of various topics: the importance of cervical screening, for instance, or the benefits of HRT. I wanted to use my experience as a clinician to empower women with knowledge, to encourage them to get to know their bodies and to dispel the myths that were often perpetuated within the area of women's health. To communicate these important messages in the most effective manner possible, I took great care to use clear language, factual terminology and evidence-based data. Furthermore, as someone with Pakistani heritage, I was keen to reach out to a South Asian audience, so I produced content in Urdu and Punjabi as well as English.

My tweets, TikTok and Instagram posts began to gather momentum and soon caught the attention of the BBC. In May 2019, they invited me onto the show to discuss the common symptoms of menopause and my efforts to raise awareness in the ethnic minority community. This appearance by a 30-something, hijab-wearing Muslim woman caused quite a stir, not just because I was talking openly about night sweats and vaginal dryness – considered taboo subjects by many – on a flagship TV programme, but also because GPs who looked like me were rarely seen on TV. The positive feedback I received as a consequence – especially from women of colour – completely blew me away.

More TV appearances followed (including on ITV) and my social media hits skyrocketed. I received thousands of responses from people across the globe who had watched one of my videos, recognized their own symptoms and – armed with new-found information – had checked in with a healthcare professional. As a GP this was music to my ears, of course, but it also highlighted a huge demand for clear, factual and accessible advice. And that, in a nutshell, is what prompted me to grab my laptop and write *The Knowledge*.

I want to share my expertise. I want to start a conversation. I want you to understand your body, to identify any changes and to realize when – and how – to seek help. Ultimately, I want you to look after yourself in the best way possible so you can lead a long, happy and healthy life. It is so important to me that women of all ages are able to advocate for themselves and get the best healthcare possible. So this series of books will cover women through every stage of life, from Puberty, to their Fertile Years, into Midlife and beyond. However, there are some elements of female health that truly do transcend the ages – I'm thinking of the need to understand your body, know your rights, and be aware of lifelong health checks.

So, this essential information is included at the front of all books in this series – to provide a comprehensive guide to female health at every stage of life.

I firmly believe that everyone assigned female at birth, regardless of age, should learn about the three distinct phases and the changes they embrace. Indeed, during the writing process I found it helpful to view things from the perspective of my 14-year-old self. I was raised in a traditional, religious Muslim household where women's health matters were hardly discussed, so I had to use other means to learn about things like menstruation and contraception. The teenage 'me' would have undoubtedly appreciated a book like this, as it would have given me a deeper understanding of myself . . . and a deeper understanding of my mother and grandmother!

And while I want to help women and girls of all ages, I'm just as keen to help their loved ones, too – that's mums, dads, siblings, grandparents and other relatives or caregivers. I particularly want to reach out to fathers, perhaps those who are single, separated or widowed – or in same-sex relationships – who may not have female partners to consult. It's so important that you feel comfortable talking to your daughters about period products, or family planning, and can do so openly and honestly.

Removing the shame and stigma from women's health is an ongoing mission of mine and forms a central theme of these books. The embarrassment factor can prove to be fatal, quite literally, if it prevents someone from getting the right care at the right time. Gynaecological cancers claim thousands of lives each year but, by performing self examinations of your breast tissue, vulva and vagina – and having regular smear tests – any changes or anomalies may be spotted early enough for you to obtain successful treatment. We also need to encourage our children and young people to familiarize themselves with their genitals without feeling ashamed. By normalizing these matters – girls checking their vulvas, boys checking their penises – good habits will be formed and infection and disease may be averted. So much of my work as a GP involves this kind of preventative care; it genuinely does save lives.

This series also offers help and advice for individuals who don't fit the mould of what society – and the healthcare system – still deem as 'normal' (although I always question this concept, because in medicine there's no such thing as a 'normal' period, for example, or a 'normal' menopause). I'm very proud of the fact that this book includes guidance for trans people and those with disabilities. These individuals have exactly the same rights to sexual and reproductive healthcare as any other patient, and should receive treatment without discrimination or prejudice. This content may also be useful to fellow clinicians, who should be ensuring their surgeries and consultations are as inclusive and as accessible as possible.

I apply a similar principle to people struggling with infertility or baby loss, whose circumstances should never be overlooked or underplayed. Successful conception, pregnancy and childbirth is still very much part of the common narrative, meaning that those who encounter problems often feel excluded from the conversation. Many women of colour can feel side-lined, too; institutional racism, combined with systemic misogyny, continues to prevail in the healthcare sector and I still hear appalling stories from women of colour whose symptoms are dismissed and whose pain is invalidated. I'm determined to combat this, and will continue to call for allies to fight our corner and for ambassadors to connect with communities.

And let me be clear: should anyone query why inclusivity, diversity and ally-ship is so important to me, and why it forms such an intrinsic part of my ethos (and this book), I'll always flip it around to ask, 'Well, why shouldn't it be important? And why should the question even need to be asked in the first place?' As far as I'm concerned, the basic principles of medicine are universal. Gold-standard healthcare should be available to all. No one should face bias or exclusion; on the contrary, they should all have a place at the table.

As a member of an ethnic group, and an employee of the UK's National Health Service (NHS), the issue of representation really matters to me. It's a known fact that most promotional healthcare material – leaflets, posters, diagrams and illustrations – does not always feature people of colour. This, quite understandably, can send the wrong signals to people who may already feel excluded from mainstream medicine, and who are therefore less likely to engage with clinicians. I'm doing my utmost to challenge and change this, and am immensely proud of the illustrations that have been specially created for this book. I only wish they'd existed when I was younger; back then, public health messaging was distinctly white, Western and middle class.

I'm also keen to break down the cultural barriers that prevent women of colour from accessing the care they need. Many of their health issues, including menstruation and menopause, are kept 'under the veil' (not spoken about, in other words), which can have a severe impact on their wellbeing. To these people – and to anybody else who's feeling alone and isolated – I truly hope I can help you to find your voice and start that conversation.

But along with being heard, you also need to feel seen. And as someone who eats, sleeps and breathes clinical medicine, I want all women to know that I see them, whether suffering with endometriosis, living with perimenopause, coping with infertility, struggling with gender identity, or simply wanting to be sure that their periods are normal. This book, I hope, will empower you to get the healthcare you deserve and, not only that, will encourage you to spread the word and tell your story. Your knowledge is a gift, to be shared freely with others. I hope this book plays a role in providing a pillar of support on that journey. You may not find every single answer within these pages – medicine is rarely one-size-fits-all, and no two people experience the same symptoms – but if you spot a nugget of advice that prompts you to pick up the phone to your doctor, or encourages you to perform your first self examination, then this labour of love will have served its purpose.

Finally, each one of us carries a candle of knowledge. Kindled by wisdom and experience, it brings light, warmth and energy. But we shouldn't keep the candle to ourselves. We should use it to light somebody else's. That way, the flame continues to burn brightly.

With love,

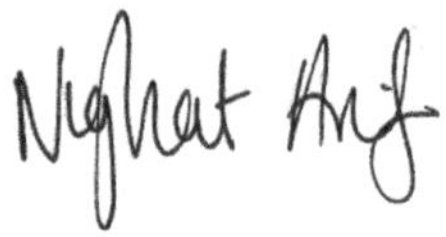

Dr Nighat Arif

Dear body, thank you for harbouring me, making me beautiful, nourishing me, making me capable of remarkable things. I promise to love and respect you.

FEMALE ANATOMY & SELF EXAMINATIONS

Awareness of your own body is key to good health, so it's vital that you educate yourself about your basic anatomy, both internal and external. In every book in this series, I have included the following pages with diagrams of the internal female reproductive system and breasts, as well as a diagram of the external vulva and pubic area. These should really help as a reference point for many sections of the book that follow.

While much of your internal anatomy won't be visible to you, it is still vital that you have a keen awareness of how areas of your body look and feel – because every body is different, only you can know your own body best. If I had my own way, every woman or person assigned female at birth (AFAB) would examine their breast tissue and genitals on a regular basis from the age of 13. Ideally, by the time you are 18, you should complete all self examinations once a month, in between periods. The more we learn about the way we look, and the way things feel, the more likely we'll be to notice changes and spot anomalies. Flagging up any concerns to your doctor may help them recognize certain symptoms and make early (sometimes life-saving) diagnoses. Pages 19–23 and 31–5 will show you how to undertake these self examinations in detail.

The female reproductive system

The female reproductive system includes everything involved in creating and carrying a baby, but it is so important to have an awareness of your system at every stage of your life, even if you never intend to have a pregnancy. The system begins at the vulva, the external element that you can see in your self examination (see pages 14–15), then moves into the vagina and then the cervix, which is the opening to the uterus. The uterus is lined with the endometrium and is where, if you are pregnant, the foetus will grow and be supported throughout your pregnancy. If you are not pregnant, then your menstrual cycle runs through a process of thickening the endometrium and then shedding the lining with your period. The ovaries are where an egg (ovum) matures each month, which is then released into the fallopian tube to travel along towards the uterus.

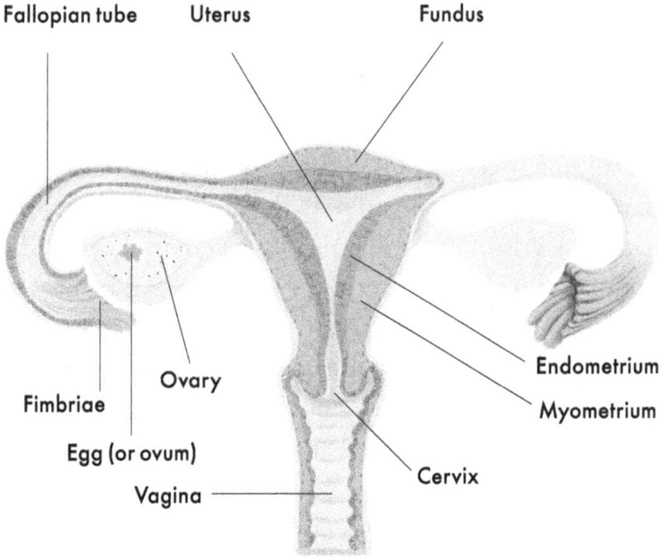
Fallopian tube
Uterus
Fundus
Endometrium
Myometrium
Ovary
Fimbriae
Egg (or ovum)
Vagina
Cervix

The female reproductive system (side view)

People are frequently surprised by how close the reproductive system is to the lower part of the digestive system, but they are all snugly clustered together within the pelvis. This is particularly important to note during times when your natural levels of the hormone oestrogen drop, as this is the reason why vaginal atrophy (see page 73) can cause infections in the urinary tract. Your bladder and urethra sit just in front of your uterus and labia, while the bowel, rectum and anus sit just behind. Between the lower opening of the vulva and the anus is an area called the perineum, which can easily split or become sore if the skin becomes dry.

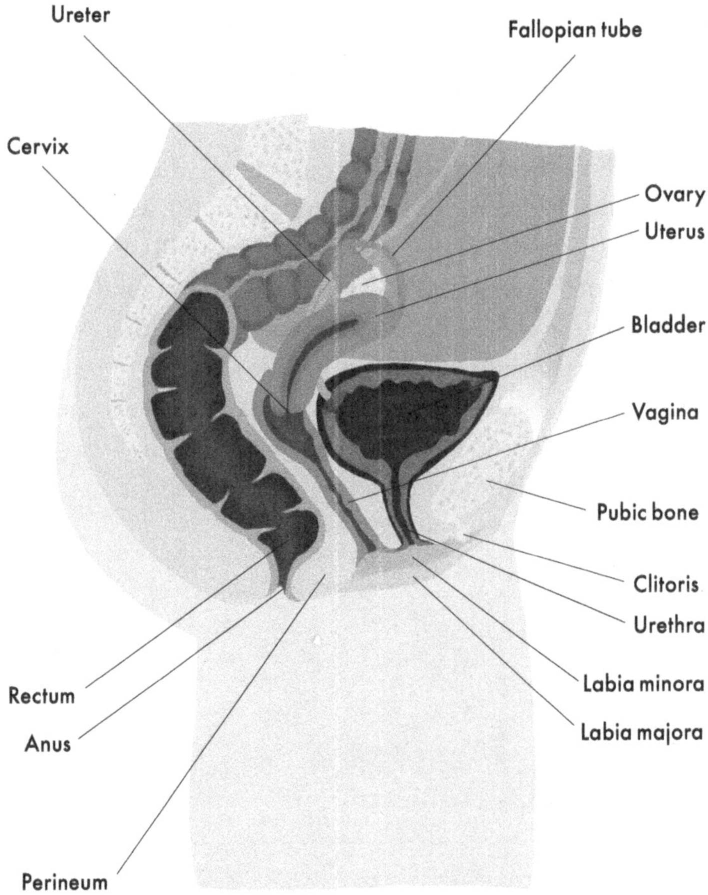
Ureter
Fallopian tube
Cervix
Ovary
Uterus
Bladder
Vagina
Pubic bone
Clitoris
Urethra
Rectum
Labia minora
Anus
Labia majora
Perineum

The vulva & pubic area

The vulva is the external part of your genitals while the pubic area is that between your legs, above your vulva, where your pubic hair grows. Looking into the vulva you will see that it's formed of the outer labia and inner labia. The clitoral hood sits at the top of the inner labia and covers the clitoris, while the urethral opening (where you urinate from) is just below. The entrance to the vagina sits at the bottom of the inner labia, then the perineum is the area of skin that sits between the openings of the vagina and the anus.

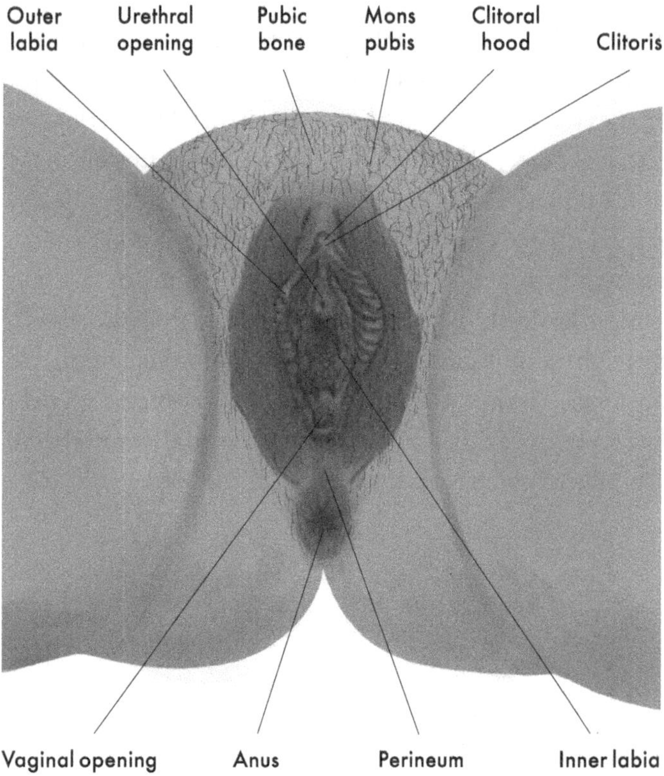
Outer labia
Urethral opening
Pubic bone
Mons pubis
Clitoral hood
Clitoris
Vaginal opening
Anus
Perineum
Inner labia

The breast

The breasts sit in front of the chest, separated from your ribs by the pectoral muscles. Each breast is formed of several lobules (or alveoli), around 15 to 20 in each breast, that are connected via milk ducts and milk reservoirs to tiny openings in the nipple. The hormonal changes associated with late pregnancy and childbirth will stimulate the alveoli to make milk and the action of a baby suckling at the breast will cause a 'let down', when the milk is released from the alveoli, through the milk ducts and reservoirs out through the nipple openings. The first milk that comes from the breast is a rich, fatty substance called colostrum and then the 'mature' milk is produced about two days after a baby is born.

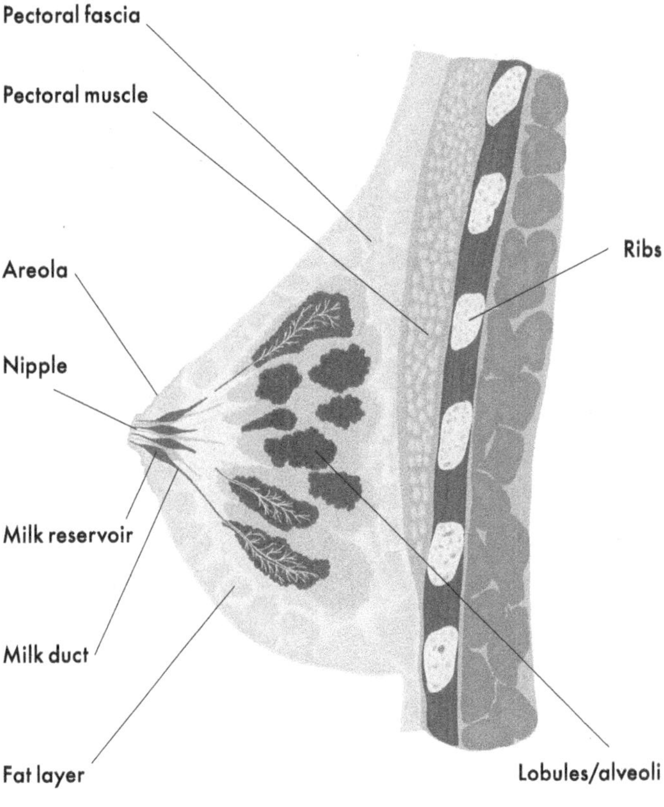
Pectoral fascia
Pectoral muscle
Areola
Nipple
Milk reservoir
Milk duct
Fat layer
Ribs
Lobules/alveoli

SELF EXAMINATION: BREASTS

Breast cancer is very common and, in the UK, about one in seven women will be diagnosed with it in their lifetime. Early detection significantly improves the chance of successful treatment and recovery, which is why it is so important to examine your breast tissue on a regular basis. Thanks to the increased raising of awareness throughout the NHS – and the fabulous work of charities like Breast Cancer Now – more women are examining their breast tissue than ever before. A thorough self examination should take about ten minutes and might just save your life.

Examining your breasts

I advise my patients to do breast examinations on a monthly basis: on roughly the same date each month, or two weeks before or after your period if you're menstruating (as fluctuations in oestrogen around your period are likely to cause breast pain and swelling that might mean missing any lumps).

Perform your breast exam wherever it feels comfortable (preferably somewhere nice and quiet, where you won't be disturbed) – perhaps on your bed, or in the bath or shower. I often tell my patients to do it at a particular time of day, which might help to jog their memory and make it a routine, perhaps in front of their bedroom mirror as they're getting dressed for work on a Monday morning. I know some women who ask their partners to have a good feel of their breast tissue – you'd be surprised how many lumps are found by loved ones – and you can always return the favour by assisting with their personal examinations. It's important to point out that those assigned male at birth can get breast cancer too, so it's a good idea for them to check their pecs regularly.

Breast implants can make a self examination more difficult but it is still important. You should be able to gently shift the position of the implant and you can then palpate around the implant to feel the breast tissue around it.

What to look out for during a breast self examination

- A new lump in the breast or armpit area, which may or may not cause pain.
- Irritation, redness, darkening or flaking of the skin around the breast and nipple area.
- A swelling or thickening in any part of the breast.
- Skin snagging, puckering or dimpling around the nipple area.
- Nipple discharge or blood if not pregnant or nursing.
- A marked and visible change in breast size (it's common for women to have one breast bigger than the other, but watch out for *recent* changes).
- A dull or sharp pain in any area of the breast.

Try to focus and concentrate as you feel your breasts. Don't be half-hearted or absent-minded! Remind yourself that you're feeling for lumps and bumps in the breast tissue and armpit area, and are looking for any changes in the skin or nipple.

If you *do* notice any irregularities during a self examination, try not to panic or assume the worst. Make a note of these changes, however small, and book an appointment to see your doctor as soon as possible, outlining the reasons to the receptionist when you call.

Do not delay matters or tell yourself that you're worrying unnecessarily. The sooner you get seen by a clinician, the better. And – should anything require further investigation – you'll be promptly referred to a specialist.

How to examine your breasts

Examine your breast tissue monthly, preferably between your periods. Find somewhere you are comfortable, either standing up or lying on your back. Then remove your top and bra. Complete the following steps on both sides.

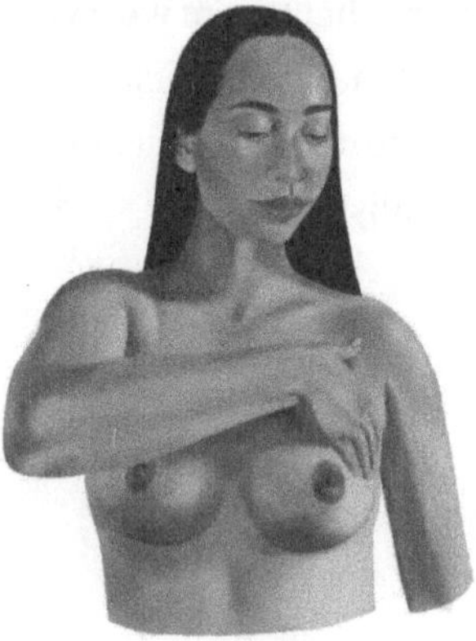

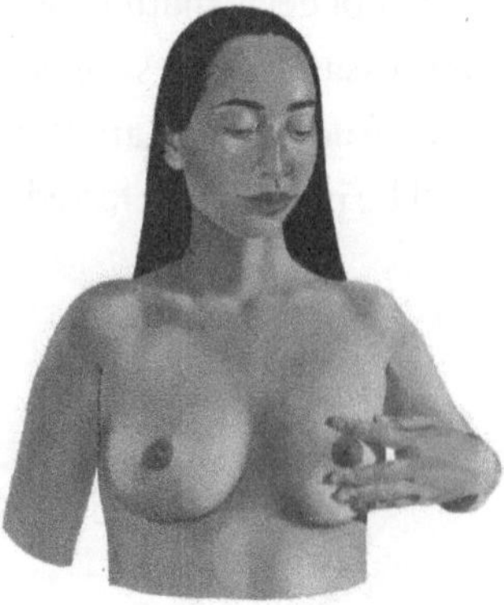

1 With the pads of four fingers, slowly press around the fleshy breast tissue in a circular motion, moving outwards from the nipple to your rib and armpit areas. Apply pressure that's firm, but comfortable. Feel for any changes to the flesh or skin as outlined opposite.

2 Use your fingers to feel underneath and around the nipple, looking for any changes to the flesh or skin.

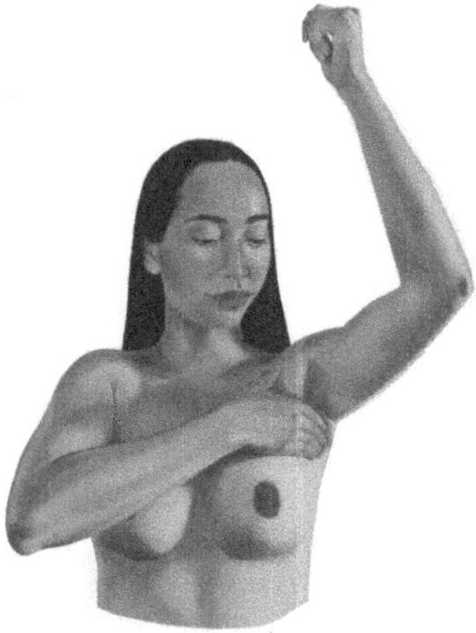

3 Use your fingers to feel underneath the armpit, looking for any changes to the flesh or skin.

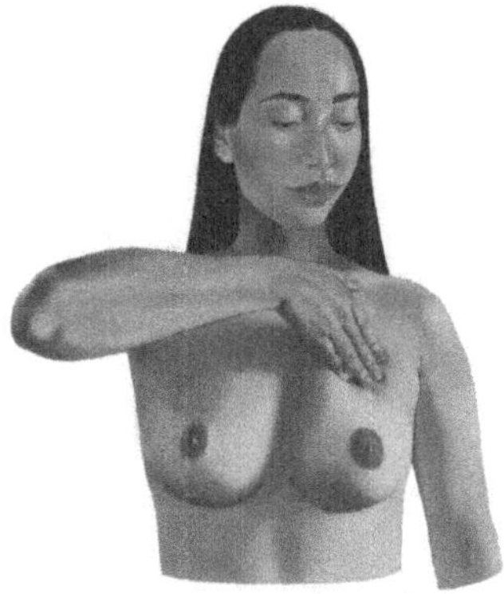

4 Walk your fingers up your chest towards your neck, feeling as you go, looking for any changes to the flesh or skin.

WEAR THE CORRECT SIZE BRA!

I see so many women in my surgery with chronic breast pain who are clearly wearing the wrong-sized bra. When I was younger, I never received any guidance about the importance of wearing the right bra. I was none the wiser until the age of 23, when a lovely lady in the lingerie department of a local shop introduced me to the joys (and comfort) of wearing a correctly fitted bra!

The easiest way to find your bra size is to visit the lingerie section of your local department store, or a stand-alone lingerie store. The staff there will be specially trained in measuring busts. Many bra-fitters now determine your size on sight, without a tape measure – a real specialist skill! If, however, you don't feel comfortable visiting a store, or can't find the time to, then you can measure yourself at home, and calculate your bra size from there.

How to measure your bra size

You'll need to take two measurements to determine your bra size: the band measurement and the cup measurement. If possible measure in inches (because that's how bra sizes are calculated), but you can use an online calculator to convert from centimetres if your tape measure doesn't show inches.

To find the band size, measure all around your ribcage just beneath your breasts. (If the measurement is an odd number then scale up or down to the nearest even number.)

This number is your band size. Then measure all around the widest area of your bust, so the tape measure sits firmly but comfortably. Subtracting your band size from this bust measurement will give your cup size, so less than 1 inch (2.5cm) = AA, 1 inch (2.5cm) = A, 2 inches (5cm) = B, 3 inches (7.5cm) = C, 4 inches (10cm) = D, 5 inches (12.7cm) = DD, 6 inches (15.2cm) = E, 7 inches (17.8cm) = F, 8 inches (20.3cm) = FF, 9 inches (22.9cm) = G, 10 inches (25.4cm) = GG, 11 inches (27.9cm) = H. Sizes beyond H are usually available from specialist retailers.

What to look for in a well-fitting bra

- It should be snug when on the loosest hook.
- The shoulder strap should sit comfortably to prevent shoulder pain.
- The cups should be flush with your bust.
- The centre wire or fabric should sit flat against the chest wall; if it pulls away the cup is not deep enough, and if it wobbles the cup is too deep.
- At the sides, the bra wire or fabric should sit under the breast along the ribs; if it sits on the breast tissue, the cup is too small, and if the side wire is too big it will dig into the underarm area.

Cup size = measurement 1 minus measurement 2

How to measure your bra size

Find somewhere you can measure yourself comfortably without being distracted, then either measure over a soft (non-padded) bra – whichever bra you currently find most comfortable to wear – or against your bare breasts.

1 Measure the circumference around the fullest part of your breasts (shown by the solid line in the image on page 29). The tape measure should have a little give in this measurement.

2 Measure the circumference around your ribcage beneath your breasts (shown by the dotted line in the image on page 29). The tape measure should be very snug, but still comfortable for this measurement.

3 Calculate your bra size using the formula on page 26.

WEAR THE CORRECT SIZE BRA!

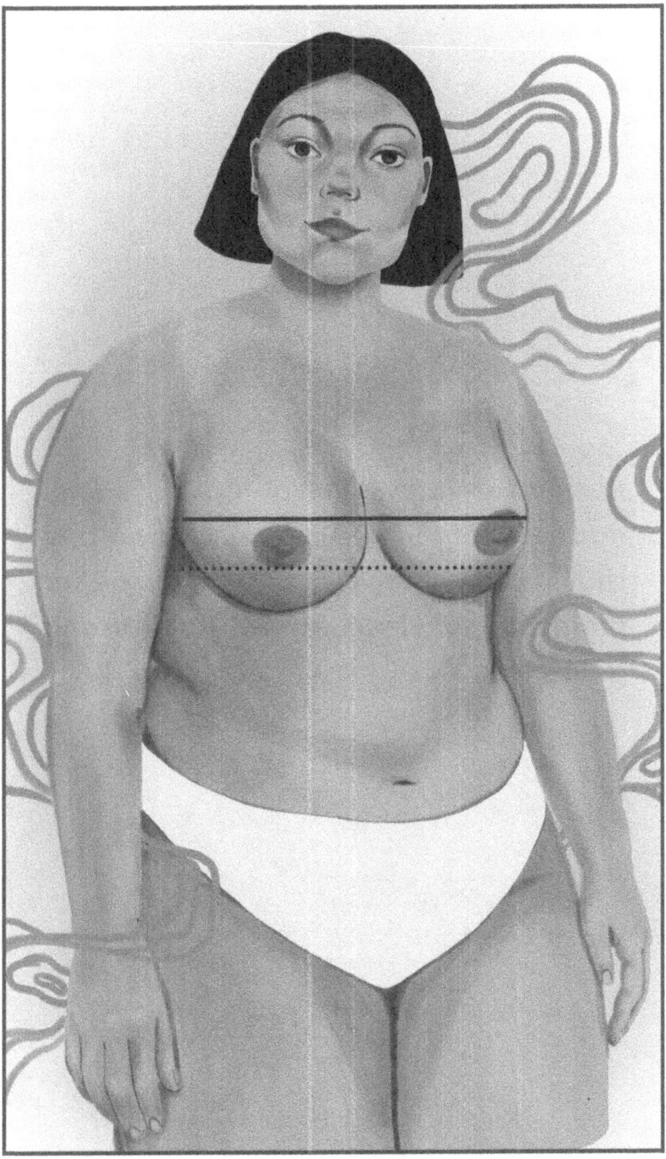

Remember: no two vulvas look the same, each is completely unique. And no one should know your vulva and vagina better than you. So why not grab a mirror and get started?

SELF EXAMINATION: VULVA & PUBIC AREA

Whilst breast self examinations have become commonplace – and have saved countless lives – there is still a huge lack of awareness around genital self examinations. This simply has to change if we are going to reduce the incidence of vaginal and vulval cancers, so it is vital you familiarize yourself with your vulva and pubic area.

Examining your vulva & pubic area

Vulval and vaginal cancers are rare but frequently missed or misdiagnosed. They can occur in women of any age, more often among those who are long-term smokers or who have a family history of melanoma (a type of skin cancer). There are 1,400 new cases of vulval cancer each year in the UK and five every week of vaginal cancer. While they are awful diseases, if picked up early, then the prognoses are encouraging. Self examination is key and, as per usual, this is a euphemism-free zone, so no talk of foo-foos or front bottoms whatsoever!

Not to be confused with the vagina, the vulva is another name for your external genitals, namely the labia majora (outer lips), the labia minora (inner lips) and the clitoris. Speaking as a doctor who has examined thousands of women, I can assure you that no two vulvas look alike.

Becoming familiar with the way your vulva looks and feels is very, very important.

If we're going to raise awareness about vulval examinations, however, we first have to remove the stigma and take away the sexualization of women's bodies in today's society. Examining and touching your vulva for health purposes isn't remotely pornographic – it's a sensible thing to do, not a sexual thing to do – and we need the men in our lives to respect and support us in this regard.

We also need to reach the stage where we can encourage our children to regularly examine their genitals without embarrassment. By normalizing things – girls checking their vulvas every week, boys checking their penises and testicles – good habits will be formed and infections and diseases may be recognized and treated at an early stage.

A vulval examination should ideally take place monthly: on roughly the same date each month, similarly to a breast examination (I often encourage my patients to get into the routine of doing the examinations one after the other). You'll need some privacy – and won't want interruptions, of course – so perhaps choose a locked bathroom or bedroom, preferably with some natural light. Find yourself a small hand-held mirror, and set aside ten minutes or so.

What to look out for during a vulva & pubic region self examination

- Any lumps, bumps, spots or sores that could indicate infection, disease or other conditions.

- Any changes to the colour or size of different areas from one examination to the next.
- Any bad-smelling discharge (though some discharge is normal, and the amount will depend on what point you are at in your menstrual cycle). If your discharge has a bad smell or is an unusual colour (see *The Power of Puberty & Periods*) it could indicate an infection.

How to examine your vulva & pubic region

Examine your vulva monthly, preferably between your menstrual periods, if you have them. Before you begin, wash your hands with soap and water, then grab a hand-held mirror and find somewhere with enough space to sit, squat or lie down, on the floor or on a chair, and sufficient light for you to see well, where you won't be interrupted for ten minutes.

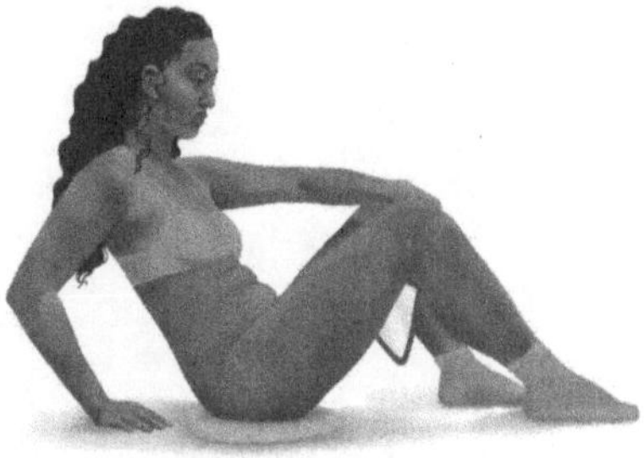

1 Open your legs and check the area where your pubic hair grows. Feel around with your fingers and position your mirror to check for moles, bumps, spots, warts, ulcers, lesions, rashes or white patches. Make a mental note of anything that looks new or feels different. Examine the fleshy area from top to bottom.

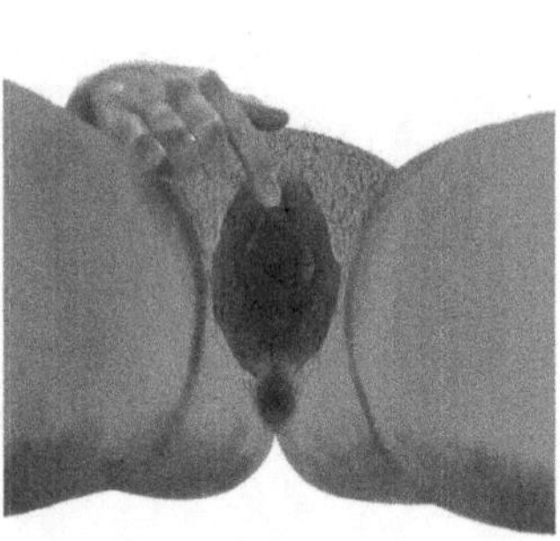

2 Next, find your clitoris – at the top of the vulva, the fold of skin where the inner labia meet – and look for any bumps, growths or discolouration.

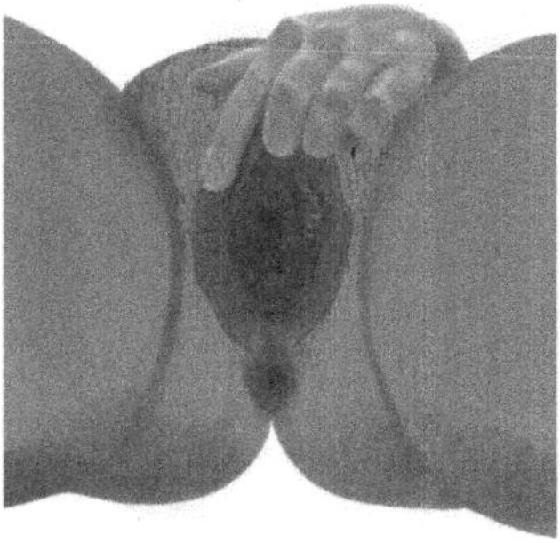

3 Check your labia majora – the outer lips – and, again, feel for any bumps, spots, lesions or rashes.

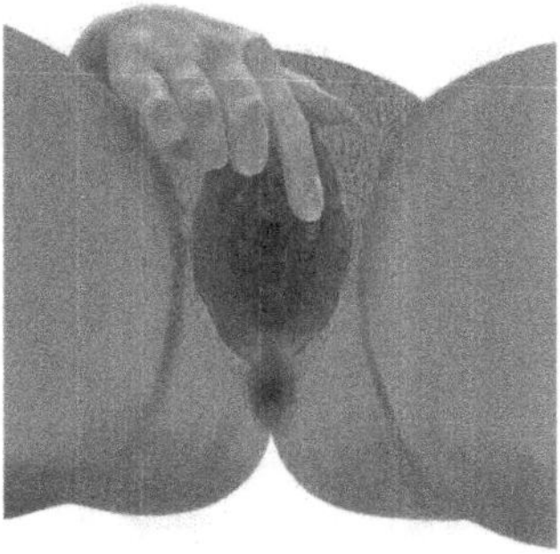

4 Check your labia minora – the inner lips – and, again, feel for any bumps, spots, lesions or rashes.

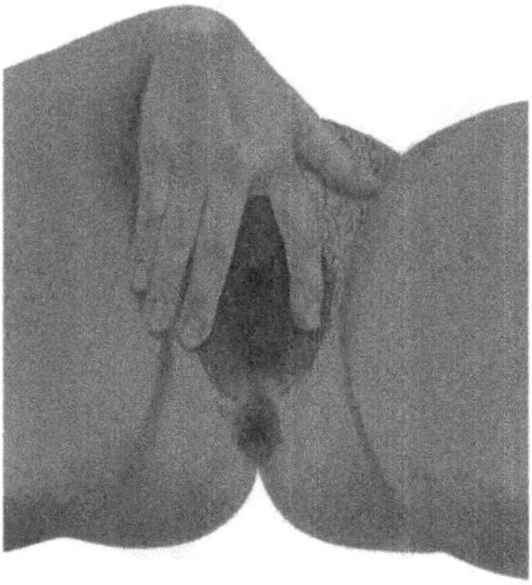

5 Prop the mirror in front of you and use one hand to gently hold open your labia minora, to see into your vagina. Check your vagina for any bumps, spots, lesions or rashes. You may see what look like 'rings' going around the vaginal wall – this is called mucosal tissue and is completely normal.

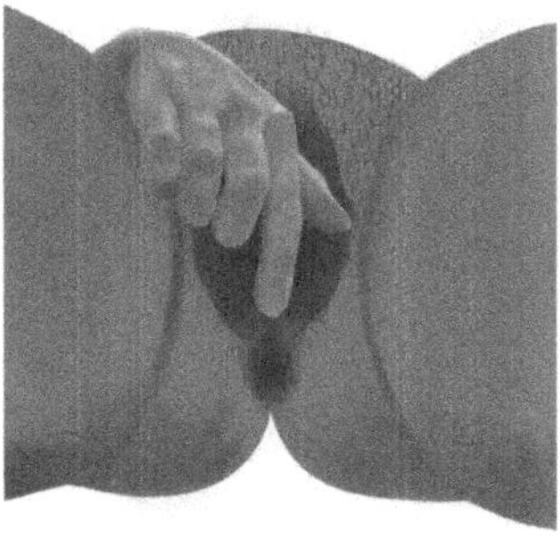

6 Finally, check your perineum (the area located between the entrance to the vagina and the anus) for any lumps, bumps or anomalies. When you have finished, wash your hands again. Make a note of any changes detected and, if you're at all worried about any anomalies, don't hesitate to consult your doctor for a professional examination.

FAIR HEALTHCARE ACCESS FOR ALL

I feel strongly that everybody – whatever their creed, colour, background, ability or gender expression – should have equal access to healthcare when they visit my surgery or any other service in the healthcare system.

However, this is still not the case for many people trying to access healthcare and advice. Patients can be discriminated against for many reasons and access to fair healthcare for ethnic minorities, those who are disabled and the LGBTQ+ community is woefully below the ideal standard. In order to counterbalance this, and to ensure that such disparity and discrimination is eradicated, we need allies to help fight our corner, and ambassadors to try to connect with our communities.

ETHNIC MINORITIES

Institutional racism and systemic misogyny continue to prevail in healthcare, to the detriment of ethnic minority women. The health issues of women of colour are often dismissed by clinicians or their own community, and their pain is downplayed and invalidated.

In some ethnic minority communities, when someone is unwell they're more likely to have a mindset of 'I will be cured if I pray hard enough' or 'this is a test of my faith'. This can lead to a reticence to address any symptoms with a doctor, and the shame and stigma persists. Women are also less likely to discuss women's health matters with others in their community – whether that's talking about examining themselves, or about a lump they've found – and this inhibits vital information sharing. It's really important for us to recognize this issue within ethnic minority communities, and to realize that more health advocates are needed in situ to raise awareness and strengthen messages.

I'm all too aware that, among Black and Asian ethnic minorities, there's still a lot of shame and stigma around breast examinations, for example. Within some parts of society – particularly faith-based communities – breasts are highly sexualized, prompting the mindset that they're something to keep hidden. This often deters women from checking their breasts at home, or having them examined by a doctor. Whatever their symptoms, ethnic minority women are also more likely to wait for an appointment with a female doctor which, due to sheer demand, can lead to a delay. If you have an immediate health concern you may be seen much quicker by a male doctor, who will be more than happy to offer you a chaperone, or let a friend or family member accompany you.

When you make a medical appointment, don't be afraid to state your preferences:

- If you feel uncomfortable being seen by a doctor of a particular gender, you may state your preference to the receptionist.
- Ask to bring someone with you to your appointment (a friend or family member) or, alternatively, you can put in an advance request for the surgery to provide a chaperone; this might be another health professional.

All doctor's surgeries will offer you a chaperone during an appointment if you prefer, or will let you take a friend or family member with you.

If English isn't your first language, and none of the doctors happen to speak your first language, you can ask the receptionist to book an interpreter for you or, if you prefer, take someone to the appointment who can translate for you.

Removing barriers

Language can be a significant obstacle for women whose mother tongue is Urdu or Punjabi, for example, and who are unable to see a doctor who speaks it. Talking about menopause or other women's health issues can be embarrassing enough for these patients, but saying 'my night sweats soak my sheets' or 'sex with my husband is really painful' via a family chaperone or an interpreter can be problematic. In order to address these issues, not only do we need a more ethnically diverse workforce in the healthcare sector, we also need Western-trained doctors (myself included) to recognize these cultural barriers.

A lack of understanding about women's health can prevent ethnic minority women from accessing the care they need. It's become a personal mission of mine to target more evidence-based information at these hard-to-reach communities, and I regularly post short videos and longer-form interviews and Q&As on social media. Most of my posts on TikTok, Twitter and Instagram are spoken or subtitled in Urdu and Punjabi, as I've realized that many women in those communities will respond much better to verbal rather than written information (illiteracy levels are particularly high among first-generation South Asian female migrants). My social media feeds share the same handle – @DrNighatArif – so please feel free to watch and share.

If English isn't your first language, you can ask for a translator if necessary (although you may have to be quite insistent).

Improving representation

Most healthcare-related promotional material – including many leaflets, posters and illustrations – does not feature people of colour. This can send the wrong message to ethnic minorities who feel excluded from mainstream medicine and are less likely to engage with healthcare professionals.

I'm doing my utmost to try to change this. In 2019 I worked with the Pausitivity campaign group to produce a #KnowYourMenopause poster in Urdu, specifically aimed at connecting with midlife women in South Asian communities. Being the first of its kind, the poster had a massive impact when it was distributed to doctors' surgeries and community centres across the UK. A poster was also produced in Welsh, too.

Over the last few years I've also had the privilege of appearing on TV including the BBC and ITV to discuss medical matters, often from a women's health perspective, which range from hot flushes to vaginal dryness. The response from my South Asian sisters has been overwhelmingly positive. They appreciate watching someone on TV who speaks for them and looks like them; let's be honest, there aren't many Muslim women wearing pink hijabs on national TV! There's no doubt about it . . . representation matters.

8.9% of residents of England and Wales did not have English as their main language in 2021

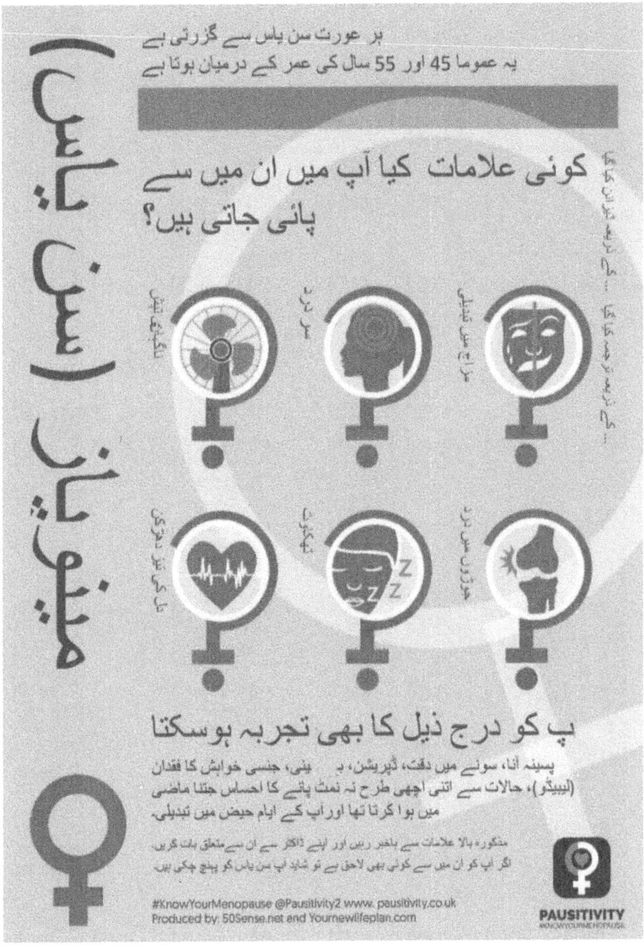

My 2019 collaboration with Pausitivity, which produced posters in Urdu to raise awareness of menopause symptoms in the South Asian community. The Pausitivity team also produced a Welsh-language poster to increase awareness in Welsh-speaking communities. Posters reproduced with thanks to Elizabeth Carr-Ellis and the Pausitivity team.

WOMEN'S HEALTH & DISABILITY

In order to reduce barriers to healthcare, doctors should make their surgeries and consultations as accessible as possible, and we should be acting as ambassadors and allies for all patients.

A 2021 article entitled 'Barriers in access to healthcare for women with disabilities' in the *BMC Women's Health* journal stated that 'women with disabilities (WWD) are more likely to have unmet healthcare needs than women without disabilities'. This statement was corroborated by the following findings outlined by the Sisters of Frida organization, a collective of disabled women:

- Disabled women have limited access to prenatal care and reproductive health services.
- Most maternity care does not meet the needs of disabled women.
- Disabled, older, asylum-seeking and Traveller women face obstacles in accessing healthcare.

In my own practice, I strive to ensure that all of my patients with physical disabilities receive the same healthcare as my able-bodied patients, and I will consider certain practicalities, such as adapting the way I fit a wheelchair user with a coil, or discussing which period products might suit their circumstances. I'll always outline the risks and benefits to an individual so they are in total control of their decision; empowering my patients is what I'm here for! If a patient is visually impaired, I'll often record voice notes, instead of writing things down or printing things out.

I also tend to use audio-based instructions for anyone who has difficulties with reading; summarizing their contraceptive options via voice notes on their phone, for instance, will always optimize healthcare for these people more than a factsheet or website. Patients with hearing loss are welcome to attend my consultations with a British Sign Language (BSL) interpreter. This is often a friend or family member but outside of this, the options are sadly limited. (A free remote interpreting service – BSL Health Access – was set up in 2020 to enable deaf people to access phone consultations but, at the time of writing, is sadly no longer funded.) Clarity of communication is vitally important when you're discussing life-changing decisions, and I hope this barrier will be removed soon.

Consultations can also be complex if I'm seeing a patient with a cognitive impairment, perhaps associated with a condition like Down's syndrome or Huntington's disease, or with neurodiverse conditions. In these instances, the way in which I communicate their healthcare options, and the way I obtain medical consent, often has to be adjusted. While I'll endeavour to involve the patient as much as possible, if they are unable to make cognitive decisions about fertility or contraception, for example, I may choose to consult with the person who has the patient's best interests at heart and who can make a decision on their behalf, often a parent, sibling or guardian.

These are just some ideas for how the healthcare system can work for all, and I hope these ideas will empower you to request the adjustments *you* may need to get the best healthcare for you, and your family too.

Become your own advocate. Get informed, do your research, become empowered and DO NOT accept discriminatory behaviour.

RIGHTS FOR TRANS PATIENTS (& ADVICE FOR THEIR DOCTORS)

Fear and apprehension can often deter trans people from seeing their doctor. This is a heart-breaking situation that can have potentially harmful consequences.

The 2018 Stonewall *LGBT in Britain Health Report* stated that, while there are 'committed individuals and organizations doing outstanding work' in the NHS and beyond, it is also true that 'instances of discrimination, hostility and unfair treatment in healthcare services are still commonplace'. Indeed, three in five trans people (62 per cent) said they'd experienced a lack of understanding of specific trans health needs by healthcare staff.

In 2021, the TransActual organization conducted their Trans Lives survey, a cross-sectional study that recorded the experiences of trans people, including those of colour and those with disabilities. Their findings were truly depressing. Fourteen per cent of respondents had been refused medical care on at least one occasion, on account of being trans. Fifty-seven per cent of trans people – that's more than half – said they had avoided going to the doctor when unwell. Fifty-three per cent of trans people of colour experienced racism while accessing trans-specific healthcare services, and 60 per cent of disabled respondents reported suffering ableism in similar circumstances.

So how can the GP experience be improved for trans

patients? Luckily, significant steps are possible to overcome those barriers and optimize their healthcare and the majority of healthcare professionals are inclusive and supportive of such adaptations and changes. The following advice, I hope, will be helpful to both patients *and* clinicians.

Changing your name & gender details

Any patient can change their name and gender on their doctor's medical records, and this can be done as an informal decision for those under the age of 16 (before they can legally change their name via deed poll). An individual can also state their preferred pronouns, whether it's he/him, she/her or they/them, for example. Surgeries should have a specific form for this purpose, which can usually be provided by the admin team. Your details will be updated on the practice IT network, and will appear on your doctor's computer screen, so there should be no need to 'explain' yourself at an appointment, which can be upsetting. More recently I've got into the habit of asking all my patients to confirm their preferred pronouns; I think it's quite an empowering thing to do.

Surgery trans policy

Ideally, your surgery will have a trans health policy and, even better, a practitioner who has a specialist interest in trans healthcare who will be best placed to understand your emotional and physical needs. For those doctors who feel their knowledge is lacking in this area – or needs updating – there are many opportunities for further learning and continual professional development and I'd like to encourage all doctors (and people!) to be aware of trans issues and how they can affect the individuals concerned.

Routine cancer screening

When a trans person changes their gender details, they are often issued with a new NHS number. It's really important to obtain confirmation from the doctor's surgery that your data has been migrated successfully so that you'll continue to receive invites for national cancer screening programmes.

Trans men, trans women and non-binary people aged 50-plus should receive an invite for a mammogram if they have breast tissue (due to either naturally occurring oestrogen or oestrogen hormone replacement). A trans man with a uterus will need to attend a cervical smear test every three years between the ages of 25 and 49, and every five years after that until they are 65.

Trans people who've changed their gender marker may not necessarily receive automatic call and recall invites for the relevant cancer screenings so please check that you've not been missed off any lists by flagging this with your healthcare provider. Ideally, there should be a member of staff with sole responsibility for keeping track of the trans patients in the recall system; my own practice has a nurse dedicated to that very task.

It's vital that trans people don't miss out on cancer screening. Double-check with your doctor that you're in the system.

Gender identity clinic referral

I hear many cases of trans people being met with ignorance, even hostility, when they've requested a referral to a gender identity, or gender dysphoria clinic (GDC), perhaps to access gender-specific counselling, medical or surgical affirming therapy, or hormone therapy. This situation requires specialist care, and patients should expect to be treated with dignity and respect before being signposted accordingly (see *The Power of Puberty & Periods* for referral options). There is also plenty of valuable guidance for doctors on the General Medical Council website, including shared care agreements and bridging prescriptions.

Shared care agreements

Some adult trans people (those over the age of 18) choose to access private healthcare for their hormone therapy – often because the waiting list for NHS clinics is so long (often years rather than months). I advise anyone doing this to diligently keep notes of your treatment as, by pursuing the private route, you are in effect becoming your own care-giver (you'll have to monitor your own blood hormone levels, for example).

You can, however, ask your GP to draw up a 'shared-care agreement' that allows an exchange of information between your private clinic and your doctor's surgery. Having these notes to hand will enable your GP to help with any issues associated with your hormone therapy, such as disrupted menstruation, clitoral growth, increased libido, increased facial and body hair (for trans men); or reduced facial and body hair, lower libido, decreased sexual function and genital shrinkage (for trans women).

Bridging prescriptions

In certain circumstances, adult trans patients who are waiting for treatment at a gender identity clinic can benefit from 'bridging' prescriptions. General Medical Council guidance currently allows GPs (preferably in collaboration with the gender identity clinic) to prescribe hormone treatment to patients who are suffering physically and/or psychologically as they wait for an appointment. In normal circumstances – outside of the bridging prescription remit – GPs are not usually expected to prescribe hormones to trans people unless they have the expertise and knowledge required.

As this has no impact on NHS budgets – hormones are relatively cheap, after all – many clinicians see this as discriminatory. My fellow GP, Dr Kamilla Kamaruddin, is a passionate advocate for trans health and is among those who find this situation problematic. When we last caught up she questioned the fact that GPs could give hormone treatment to cisgender males who had hypogonadism (a condition that can cause erectile dysfunction), the safety profile for which is similar to prescribing testosterone treatment to trans-masculine people, and GPs could also prescribe gonadotropin-releasing hormones to cisgender male patients with prostate cancer, and to cisgender females with endometriosis, but some GPs were reluctant to prescribe hormones to trans patients under a shared-care prescribing agreement with the GDC.

Complaints procedure

Each surgery has a complaints procedure. If you experience any form of intolerance or discrimination from a doctor, or a member of surgery staff, or if your GP has done nothing to help you, you should report it. You can either register a complaint with your practice manager or contact your local health authority (this advice applies to patients across the board, of course). You are also entitled to request to see a different doctor within your practice, and you can switch your surgery without having to provide a reason. Your local LGBTQ+ group may be able to suggest a more suitable alternative.

When people gain useful knowledge and information about their health issues, they'll go around sprinkling it like confetti . . .

MENOPAUSE & MIDLIFE

INTRODUCTION

Midlife – which if the average lifetime is 80 years, has arrived by your forties – should be a time to enjoy and cherish. Maybe your children are no longer getting under your feet, your career is progressing nicely and you have more quality time to spend with loved ones. Perhaps you're feeling full of energy, vigour and optimism, and are ready to embrace the future. If this sounds like you, bravo!

However, for some of us this isn't always the case. As the menopause approaches and our hormone levels naturally plummet, our quality of life can dip. We can begin to suffer problematic symptoms that affect our minds and bodies – from night sweats to vaginal dryness, and from anxiety attacks to memory fog – and, as a result, we're left feeling flat, lost and joyless.

Due to the stigma that surrounds this stage of life – together with an historical lack of knowledge and understanding within healthcare – many individuals opt to suffer in silence rather than seek help. The menopause phase is perceived as something to endure – like menstruation and childbirth – and we should just persevere regardless, perhaps not even realizing that our issues are hormone-related. As a consequence, some women can spend years living with a cocktail of debilitating symptoms, not only receiving limited support or guidance, but also missing out on beneficial treatment.

Luckily, the menopause conversation is starting to change. Awareness of the issue has skyrocketed in the UK over the past few years, largely due to dogged campaigning by healthcare pioneers like Dr Louise Newson, Diane Danzebrink, Kate Muir, Katie Taylor, Nina Kuypers, Dr Annice Mukherjee, Dr Liz O'Riordan, Lavina Mehta, Anita Powell, Meera Bhogal, Dame Lesley Regan, Karen Arthur and Sangeeta Pillai – my heroes! – as well as the sterling efforts of proactive Members of Parliament such as Carolyn Harris, Caroline Nokes and Maria Caulfield. By sharing their midlife stories with such honesty and candour, high-profile TV presenters like Davina McCall, Lorraine Kelly and Louise Minchin have also helped to break the taboo and open the dialogue. Even members of the royal family – the Countess of Wessex being a case in point – are doing their bit to shift attitudes. Menopause is normal and shouldn't be feared!

As a result of this call to arms, an increasing number of women are empowering themselves with menopause-related knowledge, and more healthcare professionals are becoming alive to their needs. I'm so proud to have played my little part in this 'revolution', too – especially within the hard-to-reach ethnic minority community that I hold so dear – and I shall continue to bang my menopause drum on TV and TikTok. Put it this way: I won't be satisfied until everyone in the UK receives the appropriate advice and treatment they need in order to lead the happy and healthy life they deserve.

THE MENOPAUSE & PERIMENOPAUSE

Everyone who menstruates will experience menopause. In purely medical terms, this is the point in life when you haven't had a period for exactly one year (you're officially deemed post-menopausal the following day). Most women reach this milestone around the age of 52 but, up to a decade prior to that, they're likely to experience what's known as perimenopause.

As women transition through life, their hormones naturally fluctuate. Levels of oestrogen dip significantly as the years pass and the ovaries are gradually depleted of functioning eggs. This perimenopausal phase can trigger numerous changes – there are well over 30 recognized symptoms – which can have a profound effect on a woman's health and wellbeing.

One in four women will sail through the perimenopausal stage without any discernible changes, and will function quite normally on a day-to-day basis. Two in four individuals will experience more significant issues that, to varying degrees, may affect their quality of life, at home, at work and beyond. Sadly, however, one in four women will endure such severe and debilitating symptoms that they'll consider taking their own life: a sobering statistic that never fails to shock me.

Most people start to have perimenopausal symptoms around the age of 40. The National Institute for Health and Care Excellence (NICE) now recommends HRT to reduce hormone-related symptoms such as night sweats and low mood (those aged 40–50 years may need higher doses of oestrogen). HRT will also help to minimize any future risk of osteoporosis and cardiovascular disease, which can be more prevalent among women suffering low oestrogen levels.

As with a woman's menstrual cycle, everyone's menopause is different. There is no one-size-fits-all template. Some women may reach menopause when they're 40, whereas others may do so over a decade later (both are perfectly normal). There's still an awful lot of confusion about the terminology, though; for years, the word 'menopause' has been used as an umbrella term for the whole midlife phase, despite the fact that, from a strictly medical perspective, it only applies to *one day* in a woman's life. The usage of the following definitions is much more accurate:

- **Perimenopause** is when you're still menstruating – even if your periods vary in flow or regularity – and having menopausal symptoms.
- **Menopause** is when you've not had a menstrual period for exactly one year, regardless of any associated menopausal symptoms.
- **Post-menopause** is when you've not had a menstrual period for at least one year and one day, regardless of any associated menopausal symptoms. You will remain post-menopausal for the rest of your life.

EARLY MENOPAUSE

Early (or premature) menopause (not to be confused with perimenopause) is diagnosed when periods stop before the age of 40. Receiving this diagnosis can be incredibly upsetting and, as fertility is affected, particularly traumatic for those who want to have children.

The causes of reaching the menopause early can be one of the following reasons.

Premature ovarian insufficiency

Known as POI, this affects one in every 100 women below the age of 40 and occurs when the ovaries stop producing hormones. We're not really sure why POI happens; it may stem from an autoimmune condition, be associated with infections like mumps, malaria and tuberculosis (TB), or there may be a familial link.

Key signs include irregular or missed periods over at least four months, with perimenopausal symptoms (see pages 67–70). A firm diagnosis is usually made after two separate blood tests, performed six weeks apart, show low oestrogen and high follicle stimulating hormone (FSH), but you may also be sent for repeat tests to track your FSH. If you are diagnosed with POI, your doctor will refer you to a gynaecologist for further investigation and treatment. For more information, see Resources from page 217.

Surgical menopause

Women (or those assigned female at birth) of any age who undergo a total abdominal hysterectomy with removal of the uterus, ovaries, fallopian tubes and cervix, can be plunged into an instant 'surgical' menopause. The removal of the ovaries results in a rapid decline in circulating oestrogen and testosterone, which means the onset of perimenopausal symptoms can be sudden and severe. Prior to surgery, women should be counselled about the risks and benefits of oestrogen-only HRT as it can regulate their symptoms. Younger patients who'd like to have children may also want to discuss the feasibility of harvesting their eggs before surgery, with a view to having children via a surrogate in the future.

Women who only have their uterus removed, and are left with their ovaries intact, are also deemed as being in surgical menopause. However, some of these patients do not realize that they're able to benefit from HRT. Years down the line, they'll come into my surgery suffering with classic perimenopausal symptoms, telling me they thought they didn't need HRT because their ovaries were still working. This can be so frustrating for all concerned.

Chemical menopause

Chemical menopause is temporary and reversible and can occur when a patient of any age is prescribed a medication called gonadotropin releasing hormone analogues (GnRHa). This drug suppresses ovulation and is used to treat PMDD (see *The Power of Puberty & Periods*) when less invasive treatments haven't worked. Some cancer treatments, such as certain breast cancer drugs, can also trigger a sudden chemical menopause. If this happens, please initiate a conversation with your doctor or your oncology team about your HRT options.

PERIMENOPAUSAL SYMPTOMS

Perimenopausal symptoms are such a mixed bag. They can range from the mild to the severe, they can ebb and flow from day to day, and they can affect different individuals in different ways. Some women may experience a handful of symptoms – maybe two handfuls – but others may not notice any changes at all. However, if you recognize any of the tell-tale signs and think you may be perimenopausal, please make an appointment with your doctor. This should ideally be a doctor who specializes in women's health, and/or who has received menopause training; don't be afraid to ask the administration team about this when you ring your surgery.

Perimenopausal symptoms could include any combination of the following:

Psychological symptoms

- Lack of self esteem
- Lack of self confidence
- Irritability
- Low mood
- Depression
- Lack of libido
- Sleep issues/insomnia
- Forgetfulness/brain fog
- Lack of focus/concentration

- Memory fog/inability to think clearly
- Verbal slips/inarticulacy

Physical symptoms

- Irregular periods
- Bladder irritation
- Urgent stress incontinence
- Dry skin
- Hair loss
- Digestive problems
- Itchy or watery eyes
- General itchiness (scalp, face, limbs)
- Change in taste
- Change in voice (rasps, wheezes)
- Mouth issues (ulcers, bleeding gums, tooth loss, nerve pain, burning mouth syndrome)
- Tinnitus
- Feeling of skin crawling/electric shocks
- Achy, heavy legs

Keep track of your perimenopausal symptoms so that you feel well-prepared if you need to consult your doctor.

'Vasomotor' symptoms

(symptoms relating to blood vessel constriction)

- Palpitations
- Headaches

- Night sweats
- Hot flushes

Vaginal & vulval symptoms

- Vaginal/vulval dryness (atrophy)
- Vaginal/vulval soreness
- Vaginal prolapse
- Recurrent urinary tract infections (UTIs)
- Difficulty having sex
- Over-lubrication
- Pain when sitting or exercising
- Discomfort during a smear test

You could also refer to the Greene Climacteric Scale (GCS), a measurement tool used by clinicians to assess symptoms with a scoring system. You can find the form online (see Resources from page 217) as it is featured on many menopause-related websites. Take the printout along to your doctor's appointment.

A note about hypermobility & hypermobility Ehlers-Danlos syndrome in perimenopause

Joint hypermobility is a genetic condition where the joints are more flexible than normal, or the joints move in excess of the normal range of motion. Joints can easily become stiff, and the condition can cause extreme fatigue. Ehlers-Danlos syndrome (EDS) – also known as hypermobility Ehlers-Danlos syndrome (hEDS) – is another genetic condition that, as well as joint-related issues, comprises a collection of symptoms that includes stretchy and/or fragile skin, poor balance and digestive problems. Many people who suffer with hypermobility and EDS are prone to migraines, but it's not commonly known that all three can be linked to the hormonal fluctuations experienced in perimenopause. If you are diagnosed with these conditions and experiencing perimenopause, the following symptoms can be heightened:

- Brain fog
- Allergies and intolerances
- Joint pain and joint looseness
- Heat intolerance

Fortunately, systemic hormone replacement therapy, or HRT (see page 121), has been shown to improve hypermobility and EDS symptoms – as well as perimenopausal migraine attacks – so, if you are experiencing these symptoms, you may want to discuss this with your doctor.

1 in 4 women said a lack of support for menopause symptoms in the workplace has made them unhappy in their job

Perimenopause is a natural transition that we should celebrate, because it means we made it to our second spring.

VAGINAL ATROPHY

Vaginal atrophy, sometimes referred to as vulvovaginal atrophy (VVA), is the thinning of the vaginal walls, which can also cause dryness and irritation. It is a common symptom of perimenopause.

Atrophy literally means 'shrinkage' and occurs when declining oestrogen levels lead to a thinning and loss of elasticity of the vaginal tissue and lining, as well as a reduction of the natural secretions that protect and lubricate the genital area. Low oestrogen levels in the bladder and urethra can also exacerbate recurrent and chronic urinary tract infections (UTIs, see *The Power of Puberty & Periods*). The bladder is situated extremely close to the vagina and so the condition can affect your bladder, too. These symptoms are particularly worsened for women affected by FGM.

It's thought that around 70 per cent of women (and those assigned female at birth) experience this progressive and chronic condition at some point in their lives. You should definitely not put up with any of these unpleasant symptoms, since effective treatment is readily available.

Symptoms of vaginal atrophy

- Dry, sore, itchy or inflamed vulva and vagina
- Pain in your bladder and/or urethra
- Recurrent UTIs
- Urgent need to urinate

- Discomfort during urination
- Very painful sexual intercourse
- Discomfort during exercise
- Discomfort and pain when sitting down
- Extreme discomfort during cervical smear test

Symptoms of VVA can range from the mildly irritating to the severely debilitating, and can significantly affect a woman's sexual health and general wellbeing. It is far more common in women over the age of 40 as they approach menopause, but it is also common among women who are breastfeeding. Self examination of the vulva and vagina can really help to pinpoint the issue before you visit your doctor; I've outlined the best way to do this on pages 31–35.

Diagnosis of vaginal atrophy

Vaginal atrophy is diagnosed by a doctor's examination and discussing your symptoms. Many affected individuals are reluctant to seek help from their doctor, often out of embarrassment or a lack of awareness. Indeed, it's estimated that less than ten per cent of sufferers receive proper care for it, often because they don't realize it's a recognized condition. This is a real shame because, with the right medication, it can be totally manageable.

Treatment of vaginal atrophy

Targeted treatment for this condition can be genuinely life-changing. People find that vulvo-vaginal itches and inflammation disappear and they go on to have the most pain-free and pleasurable sex ever! Treatments range from non-hormonal to hormonal options and you should discuss with your doctor which are best for you (see page 121).

Effects of vaginal atrophy

Vaginal atrophy is the thinning and loss of elasticity of tissue in and around the vagina and vulva. It is common in perimenopause as decreasing levels of oestrogen leads to changes to the cells and lining of the vagina. The vagina's usual size and thickness is shown opposite on the left and the thinned, less elastic vagina is shown on the right.

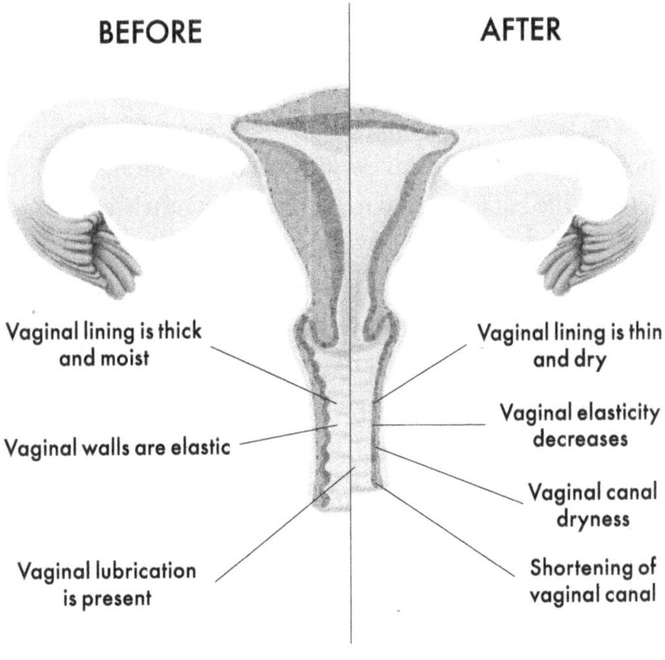
BEFORE
AFTER
Vaginal lining is thick and moist
Vaginal walls are elastic
Vaginal lubrication is present
Vaginal lining is thin and dry
Vaginal elasticity decreases
Vaginal canal dryness
Shortening of vaginal canal

Non-hormonal treatments: vaginal moisturizers & lubricants

We regularly moisturize our face, arms and legs to keep the skin plump and supple, so why not give the same TLC to our vulva and vagina, too? Readily available water-based vaginal moisturizers and gels can be used to treat and manage vaginal atrophy, and should be applied to the genital area at least every other day. These can be used during sex, too, as can oil-based vaginal lubricants.

You're never too young or too old to start using vaginal moisturizers. I would advise all women over the age of 30 to get into the habit of regularly moisturizing their vulva and vagina. By doing so they'll be maintaining good health and helping to stave off any future problems. As someone who tries to practise what she preaches, I'm happy to say that I do this at least every other day. Hyalofemme vaginal gel is another option if you prefer a gel formula.

To avoid irritating the vagina or causing infections, I would advise you to ensure your moisturizer or lubricant does not contain glycols, parabens, petroleum, perfume, flavouring, glitter, dyes or tingling ingredients. If you are prone to thrush then also avoid lubricants with glycerins.

Hormonal treatments: vaginal oestrogen

I am a *huge* fan of vaginal oestrogen – the different types and preparations are listed on pages 144–47 – and I could quite literally talk about it all day. It's a simply brilliant treatment for vaginal atrophy and, by restoring urogenital tissues, works to alleviate all those awful symptoms and provide life-long relief. Vaginal oestrogen has no side effects and is completely safe to use, either on its own or in conjunction with other HRT regimes.

Since it contains tiny amounts of hormones (not enough to enter the bloodstream) and just treats the localized vaginal area, vaginal oestrogen does not carry the risks of systemic forms of HRT. It can even be used by patients who currently have breast cancer or who have previously had breast cancer as it does not worsen breast cancer or cause a recurrence. This means that it can be prescribed for women who have (or have had) oestrogen-receptor positive breast cancer. You can also use vaginal oestrogen without progesterone, even if you have a uterus, as the hormone levels are so low.

Some brands of topical vaginal oestrogen act as a lubricant as well as hormonal treatment, therefore they can be used by women whose vulvo-vaginal pain or atrophy may be related to episiotomies, sexual trauma, birth trauma or some cases of female genital mutilation (FGM).

A note on urinary tract infections caused by vaginal atrophy

Recurrent urinary tract infections (UTIs) are very common during the perimenopause and post-menopause, as they can be exacerbated by declining levels of oestrogen. To tackle these UTIs, women are often prescribed antibiotics by their doctor in the first instance. However, when these infections are frequent, patients can develop a resistance to repeated courses of antibiotics, and this can spiral into life-threatening sepsis. Research has shown that vaginal oestrogen can often be a more effective long-term solution to prevent UTIs from occurring by keeping the vaginal walls plump and lubricated and therefore preventing the irritation that can lead to a UTI.

External vulval atrophy

Vulval atrophy is the thinning and loss of elasticity of tissue in and around the vulva and usually occurs alongside vaginal atrophy. It is common in perimenopause as decreasing levels of oestrogen leads to changes to the cells and lining of the vulva. The vulva's usual size and thickness is shown opposite on the left and the thinned vulva is shown on the right. The thinning and accompanying dryness of vulval atrophy can lead to generalized soreness of the vulva.

VAGINAL ATROPHY

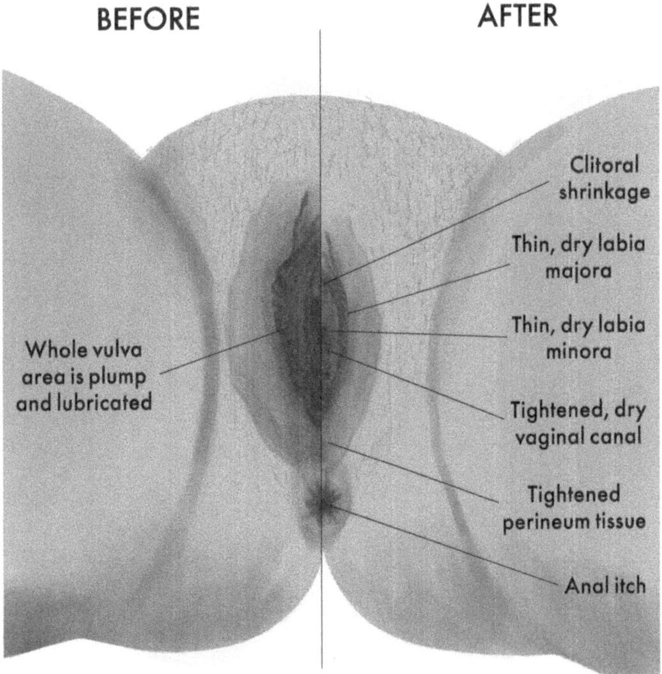
BEFORE
AFTER
Whole vulva area is plump and lubricated
Clitoral shrinkage
Thin, dry labia majora
Thin, dry labia minora
Tightened, dry vaginal canal
Tightened perineum tissue
Anal itch

URINARY INCONTINENCE & BLADDER CONTROL

Many women suffer with urinary incontinence and bladder control problems during the menopause phase of life.

Urinary incontinence during menopause is thought to be caused by decreasing levels of oestrogen that may weaken the urethra (the 'tube' that helps keep urine in the bladder until you're ready to pee). The urethra and bladder muscles can also lose some of their strength with the natural ageing process – as is the case with most muscles – and this means you may not be able to hold in as much urine as you get older.

Incontinence can be a very distressing and debilitating condition. It can dominate every thought process, so much so that those affected find themselves planning journeys, work events or day trips based on the location of the nearest toilet. The condition can severely dent a person's confidence and self-esteem, whether it's wearing incontinence pads, worrying about smelling of urine or experiencing leakages during intercourse.

Urinary incontinence impacts one in three women – so if it affects you, you're not alone – and it certainly isn't just an older person's ailment. The condition is not a laughing matter either and, instead of being ridiculed, those impacted should be treated with care and compassion, from doctors recommending tailored treatment to employers offering regular toilet breaks.

Types of incontinence & their symptoms

- **Urge incontinence** leads to urine leaks when you have a strong urge to wee or when you can't make it to the bathroom in time.
- **Stress incontinence** leads to leaks when you cough, sneeze, laugh or exercise, as these actions increase stress on the bladder and pelvic floor muscles.

Diagnosis of urinary incontinence

Urinary incontinence is easily diagnosed by keeping track of your symptoms with your doctor.

Treatment for incontinence

- **Vaginal oestrogen HRT** (see page 128) can improve symptoms of both urge and stress incontinence.
- **Vaginal pessaries** (see *The Power of Female Health, Fertility & Pregnancy*) can be prescribed by your doctor to help reduce symptoms of stress incontinence.
- **Medications** can be prescribed to help with incontinence, including solifenacin, tolterodine and mirabegron. These work by relaxing the muscles around the bladder, helping to increase the volume of urine the bladder can hold and control the release of urine.
- **Referral to a urogynaecological** specialist (who can give treatments including Botox™ injections into the

bladder) may be possible for some patients, although this is often subject to a postcode lottery.

Pelvic floor rehabilitation

I recommend that everyone performs 'squeeze and lift' pelvic floor contractions on a daily basis (see page 88) whether or not you suffer with urge or stress incontinence. If you do have symptoms, though, I suggest you gradually try to work towards completing ten long and ten short contractions, three times a day, but if you have no symptoms then once a day is sufficient. Don't over-exert yourself; just take things easy at first, and do what feels comfortable for you. You may also consider reducing your intake of caffeine, alcohol, fizzy drinks and citrus drinks, which are all thought to irritate the bladder.

Ideally, pelvic floor rehabilitation should be done in partnership with a physiotherapist who specializes in that area. You can ask your family doctor for a referral to an NHS physio (who may be based at a local continence clinic) but, again, availability very much depends on your local NHS service provision. Alternatively, you can book yourself in with a private practitioner.

A specialist physiotherapist will tailor a programme of exercises that are right for you, as well as recommending other helpful techniques to help control your bladder leakage. This may include 'the knack' – also known as the counter bracing technique – which is a method of tightly contracting your pelvic floor muscles immediately before a cough, sneeze or laugh.

Pelvic floor exercise

The 'squeeze and lift' pelvic floor contractions shown opposite will help to tone and strengthen the muscles of your pelvic floor, which in turn can lessen urinary incontinence. Repeat the exercise for ten long contractions (holding each for ten seconds) and ten short contractions (contracting and relaxing in rapid succession), up to three times a day.

1 Squeeze and lift the muscles at the bottom of your pelvic floor, and at the front and back of your tummy, as if you are trying to hold in urine mid-flow. Hold for ten seconds for long contractions and release immediately for short contractions.

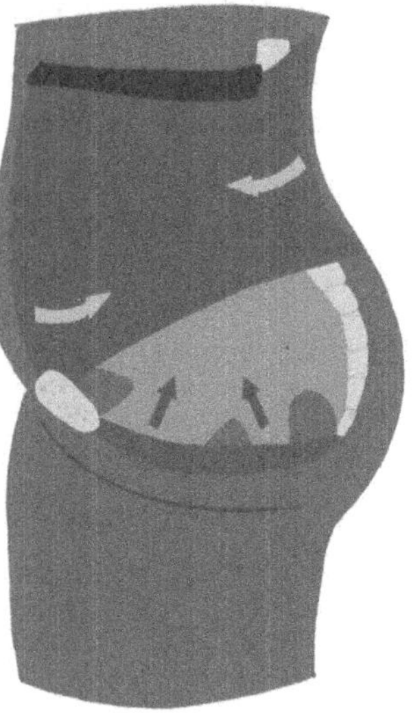

2 Release the muscles and relax while keeping your posture straight. Repeat these long contractions ten times and then repeat the exercise as ten short contractions.

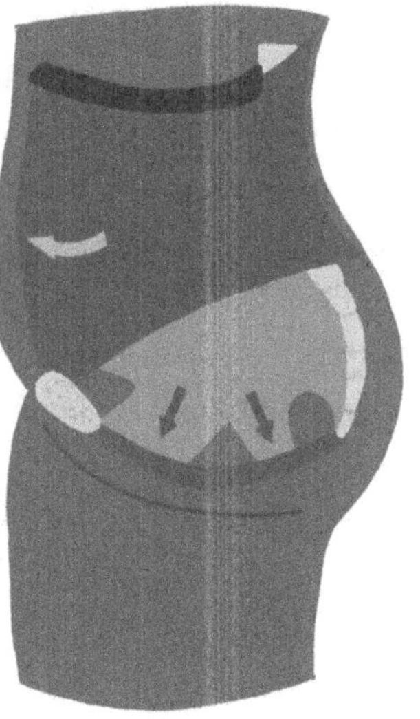

Permimenopause & contraception: is contraception necessary?

There's a great deal of misunderstanding and misinformation about midlife contraception, so let's first focus on a couple of key facts. Firstly, if you're still having periods – with or without menopausal symptoms – you can still get pregnant. Your eggs can still be fertilized by sperm so you will need to use contraception. Secondly, although some women use the coil as the progesterone element of hormone replacement therapy (see page 148), no other forms of HRT act as a contraceptive! Taking HRT may help to treat your perimenopausal symptoms, but it does not prevent you from becoming pregnant, unless you are using the Mirena™ IUS coil as part of your HRT.

So when can you safely stop using contraception? Here are the guidelines from the NHS:

- **Continue to use contraception for two years** after your last menstrual period if you're under 50 years of age.
- **Continue to use contraception for one year** after your last menstrual period if you're over 50 years of age.
- **Continue to use barrier methods of contraception** (such as condoms) to protect yourself from sexually transmitted diseases, regardless of your age. Contrary

to popular belief, STDs can be caught and passed on at any age; according to the charity Age UK, between 2014 and 2018 there was a 23 per cent increase in STD diagnoses among men and women in the 65-plus age bracket.

MIDLIFE SEX ISSUES

There is absolutely no reason why you shouldn't be enjoying a healthy and active sex life well into your middle age (in fact, for the rest of your life). Many patients of mine who are in their forties and fifties will proudly tell me they're having the best sex of their lives, without the inconvenience of monthly periods and the interruptions of young children. Not every woman is so fortunate, however, and many suffer sexual problems that lead them to avoid lovemaking altogether. The hormonal imbalances associated with perimenopause can play a huge part, since they can cause a host of physical and psychological symptoms. If this sounds like you, please don't despair; I'd urge you to talk to your doctor and discuss your options.

Lack of libido

It can feel awkward and uncomfortable to talk about your sex drive, and most of us won't like to admit that it's in decline. However, low libido is a very common issue among midlife women, and can be treated very successfully. We know that testosterone therapy can work wonders (see page 151) although, at the time of writing, obtaining a prescription can sometimes be tricky as female testosterone is not licensed on the NHS. Testosterone usually prescribed to men can be used 'off licence' in low doses for female HRT use if your NHS doctor has it initiated by a menopause specialist, or feels comfortable prescribing it themselves; the latter usually depends on their local Integrated Care Board (ICB) or Integrated Care System (ICS) marking it as 'green' on their NHS formulary (list of medicines).

There are other non-medical ways to address low libido, too, although they're not necessarily quick fixes. Eating well, minimizing stress and enjoying plenty of exercise can really help things in the bedroom; the latter in particular can boost your levels of serotonin – the so-called 'happy hormone' – and can make you feel much better about yourself. Patients of mine have often found that, by improving their general wellbeing, their sex life has benefited greatly.

Sexual dysfunction

A woman's libido can also be affected by any sexual problems her male partner is experiencing. Many men suffer with erectile dysfunction, especially as they approach middle age; this can be linked to underlying issues such as high blood pressure, type 2 diabetes or poor mental health, and often has nothing to do with a lack of intimacy or a lack of sexual chemistry. Nonetheless, erectile dysfunction is still one of those taboo subjects that men and women find really difficult to discuss, even if they've been with their partner for decades. However, as a doctor who's counselled hundreds of couples, I know how common these issues are; statistics show that about 60–70 per cent of couples have sex-related difficulties at some point in their lives. My message to you is, never feel embarrassed to talk to a health professional.

Please go and see your doctor – as a couple, ideally – and have that conversation.

Painful sex

Painful sex can be more prevalent in the menopause phase when women are more likely to suffer with vaginal atrophy. Painful sex is not talked about nearly enough, though – despite being very common – and usually stems from one or more of the following issues:

- Vaginal atrophy or genitourinary syndrome of the menopause (see page 73).
- Vulvodynia (see page 218).
- Endometriosis (see pages 211).
- Birth trauma.
- Female genital mutilation (FGM).
- Vaginismus – this is an autonomic (out of your control) reaction to the fear of vaginal penetration. Whenever penetration is attempted, the vaginal muscles tighten up. You can suffer with occasional vaginismus even if you've had painless vaginal penetrative sex in the past.

Use lube, lube and more lube for each and every vaginal or anal sexual encounter.

In order to minimize pain and discomfort during sex, I often recommend one of my favourite top tips, namely the double slide method. It takes two to tango in the bedroom, yet so many women – and trans men who still possess a vulva and a vagina – will assume that painful sex is their problem alone. Nothing could be further from the truth . . .involving your partner is actually part of the solution.

The double slide method

Before penetration, the woman applies a water-based vaginal moisturizer inside her, which is absorbed into the skin of the vulva and vagina. At the same time, their partner applies an oil-based vaginal lubricant (it has to be vaginal) onto their penis or sex toy.

Find ways of relaxing your body that work for you. Do things at your own pace, communicating what you like to your partner and perhaps showing them yourself. Don't be disheartened if your first attempt at this method doesn't go to plan; try it again on another occasion, but in the meantime keep exploring ways of maintaining intimacy that suit you best as a couple.

The double slide can be really effective due to the fact that oil and water don't mix – they slip and slide – which allows for more comfortable sex. And, since soreness and irritation can be reduced by this method, you're also much less likely to suffer with urinary tract infections (UTIs) which can be very common during perimenopause and post-menopause.

Don't always assume that your anxiety or low mood is symptomatic of depression; it could be the result of a hormonal imbalance.

PERIMENOPAUSE & MENTAL HEALTH

In midlife, many women notice that perimenopause can have a profound effect on their mental health, memories and general wellbeing.

Perimenopause can trigger a wide range of psychological symptoms, including the following:

- Memory fog
- Mood swings
- Anxiety attacks
- Lack of motivation
- Loss of confidence
- Paranoid thoughts
- Irritability
- Anger
- Sleep disturbance
- Decreased sexual interest

Some women will also experience suicidal thoughts. Global data suggests that the highest rate of suicide among women is between the ages of 45 and 54, and some studies indicate that this may be related to the biological changes experienced during perimenopause and menopause (see Resources from page 217).

Hormonal fluctuations can wreak havoc with a person's mood, leaving them angry one minute, tearful the next, and confused as to why this is happening. Affected individuals will often say the following when they see me in surgery:

'I can't cope with these meltdowns and mood swings . . . it's so out of character', 'I feel like I'm losing my mind . . . I'm so worried I've got dementia', 'I can hardly focus or concentrate on anything . . . I feel totally lost', 'All the joy has been sucked from my life . . . I've never felt so depressed'.

This can be a very isolating time, especially if a person believes they're alone in feeling this way. They might also feel an element of shame about their uncharacteristic mood swings and anger, which could deter them from opening up to friends and family. It's very important, therefore, to seek professional help sooner rather than later.

A lack of understanding about perimenopause, however, can lead to misdiagnosis. I've known cases of midlife women being told they're suffering with depression and being prescribed anti-depressants when, in many instances, their emotional and psychological issues are directly related to their changeable hormones, which can be successfully treated and regulated with HRT.

If you experience an acute mental health crisis, and are worried about your immediate safety, call 999 for urgent care.

Other than seeing your doctor, who will be happy to discuss therapies and strategies, there are alternative avenues you can pursue, including:

- **Self-refer to NHS Talking Therapies** (see Resources from page 217)
- **Text 'SHOUT' to 85258** in the UK at time of crisis and a counsellor will text you back.
- **The Samaritans charity** can be contacted by phoning 116123.
- **The Mind charity** can offer support and care for those with mental health issues.

Neurodiversity during menopause

Neurodiversity refers to a wide spectrum of human behaviour including moods, attention, sociability and learning abilities, and people across the spectrum of neurodiversity should be supported by their healthcare professionals in the best ways for them. All the above behaviours can also, however, be adversely affected by perimenopause, so it can be a particularly disconcerting time for neurodiverse people, and also a time when neurodiverse conditions, that might have been missed in earlier life, may be diagnosed.

Autism, attention deficit hyperactivity disorder (ADHD), Tourette syndrome and dyslexia are common neurological conditions and people with autism and ADHD in particular can notice a significant impact on their mental wellbeing during perimenopause.

Autism spectrum disorder

Throughout a person's lifetime autism spectrum disorder (ASD) can affect communication, behaviour, social skills, attentiveness and learning. There is currently very little research into the effects of perimenopause on individuals with ASD, but on the few studies that we do have, the common denominator indicated a significant increase during perimenopause in autism-related symptoms, such as socializing, communicating and sensory sensitivity.

Data also shows that women are generally better at 'masking' their symptoms and finding coping strategies to deal with ASD and so women have historically been underdiagnosed in comparison to men. This has had a knock-on effect in the lack of studies around the effects of ASD during perimenopause.

Attention deficit hyperactivity disorder

Commonly known as ADHD, this is a common condition diagnosed in both children and adults, that manifests in hyperactivity, difficulties paying attention and impulsive behaviour.

The reduced oestrogen levels associated with perimenopause also reduce levels of dopamine, a chemical that aids executive functioning. This means that women with ADHD can find their symptoms worsened by the hormonal changes of perimenopause, in addition to the common mental health implications of perimenopause.

One survey, by *ADDitude* magazine, found that more than half of the women surveyed said 'ADHD had the greatest impact on their lives' during the perimenopausal years from their forties to their fifties with brain fog and memory issues having the most impact. In addition, many women also report ADHD symptoms for the first time during perimenopause. If you are diagnosed with ADHD, discuss your HRT options with your doctor, as oestrogen replacement could have a significant impact on your wellbeing.

LIFESTYLE CHANGES TO HELP RELIEVE PERIMENOPAUSAL SYMPTOMS

In midlife, many women make lifestyle changes to control their perimenopausal symptoms but these will have a huge beneficial effect on their overall wellbeing, too.

Sleep

Cognitive behavioural therapy (CBT) can help with sleep issues by encouraging positive thoughts and better habits (see pages 117–120) but there are other practical things you can also do to aid a restful night:

- **Avoid eating meals late at night**, and steer clear of alcohol and caffeine.
- **Take a bath** before you go to bed.
- **Keep your bedroom cool**, dark and ventilated.
- **Place a towel beneath you** to absorb perspiration and protect your sheets.
- **Use a special cooling pad pillow** (there are plenty on the market), which can ease night sweats.
- **Wear loose cotton nightwear** that can easily be removed in bed.
- **Reduce distractions before bedtime**; maybe read a book or listen to calming music rather than watch TV or scroll social media.

- **Use a sleep app** to help you dose off (see Resources from page 217).

Diet

Maintaining a varied and nutritious diet can make a significant difference to your general health and wellbeing, and this is particularly important as you approach the menopause. Many individuals in this phase of life find themselves gaining weight – especially around their abdomen – which is often the result of the following factors:

- Fluctuating hormone levels can affect the way your body stores fat, leading to fewer calories being burned, and more fat building up.
- A decrease in muscle mass means your body may crave more calories, and you may end up eating more food than you actually require.
- You may be less inclined to take regular exercise because of perimenopausal symptoms such as insomnia, fatigue, hot flushes and joint pain.

Weight gain in the midlife years can often increase your risk of certain illnesses – such as type 2 diabetes and cancer – so it's vital that you watch what you eat and drink. I'm no fan of restricted, prescriptive diets – I much prefer sensible, achievable and balanced healthy eating plans – and my key advice to patients is as follows:

Eat lots of fruit & vegetables

Fruit and veg should form a core part of your daily diet. My esteemed colleague Dr Mary Claire Haver, a US-based obstetrics and gynaecology physician who specializes in women's nutrition, recommends eating a 'rainbow' of brightly coloured fruit and veg. So that means plenty of orange satsumas, red grapes, green peppers and purple sprouting broccoli!

Up your intake of fibre & protein

Make sure your daily food quota includes lots of high-fibre, starchy carbohydrates (such as brown rice, wholegrain pasta and baked potatoes) as well as a variety of protein-rich foods such as oily fish, lean meat, eggs, nuts, seeds and legumes (beans and pulses).

Cut down on highly processed food & junk food

Try to reduce your intake of processed foods, takeaways and ready meals. They may contain high levels of salt and saturated fat, and can lack essential nutrients. Some cured meats may also contain a preservative called sodium nitrate that has been linked to cancer and heart disease.

Eat sugary foods only in moderation

I'm not averse to grabbing a slice of cake or a bar of chocolate when I'm feeling tired or stressed. However, while I don't deny myself the occasional treat, I try not to make it a daily habit. Foodstuffs with added sugar such as sweets, cakes, biscuits and fizzy drinks – as well as those with hidden sugars, like pasta sauces and flavoured yogurts – should be consumed in moderation.

Reduce portion sizes

Your stomach is much smaller than you think – it's actually about the same size as your clenched fist (go on, try it!) – so try reducing your portion size accordingly. To prevent overeating, learn to recognize the feeling of your stomach being full, and remind yourself that you don't have to clear the entire plate.

Maintain good gut health

It's so important to keep your gut healthy. Not only does it detoxify and eliminate what we consume, it also controls our mind and body. It's responsible for managing neurotransmitters such as serotonin (the 'happy hormone'), dopamine, cortisol and melatonin, all of which affect our mood and sleep. The gut also plays an integral part in the menopause phase. We know that oestrogen, together with other hormones and toxins, gets excreted into the gut before being eventually eliminated from the body via faeces. Constipation is common in the perimenopause and post-menopause, however, and if the gut microbes become imbalanced it can lead to oestrogen absorbance dominance. This can heighten menopausal symptoms, hence why you need to look after your gut by sticking to a healthy and nutritious diet.

Consider food supplements & vitamins

In order to maintain healthy joints, skin and hair during menopause – and to look after your immune system – I generally recommend the following dietary supplements to my patients:

- Vitamins B_6, B_7 (biotin) and B_{12}
- Vitamin D
- Magnesium
- Collagen
- Zinc
- Calcium
- Omega 3 oil
- Evening primrose oil
- Soya isoflavones

Some of the above can be found in multivitamin tablets (which I recommend you take on a daily basis in any case), but others may need to be purchased separately.

81.9% of post-menopausal women have low levels of magnesium.

Eat phytoestrogens

There is also some evidence to suggest that foods high in phytoestrogens – including olive oil, soya beans, tofu, miso, liquorice root tea, beans, pulses, oats, nuts and seeds – can relieve symptoms of hot flushes and can improve bone health.

Cut down on alcohol

Not only does alcohol contain 'empty' calories, it can also worsen common perimenopausal symptoms like hot flushes, night sweats and low mood. Excessive consumption also increases your risk of cancer and heart disease, among other illnesses. If you can't eliminate it altogether, stick to the NHS recommended limit of 14 units of alcohol per week.

Healthy eating habits, drinking plenty of water, getting regular exercise and good-quality sleep can make such a difference to perimenopausal symptoms. Give yourself time for some self-care!

Drink plenty of water

I can't stress how important water is. Not only does it quench your thirst, it also helps to regulate your body temperature, lubricate your joints, ease your digestion, improve concentration and stave off infections. Staying well hydrated also aids a good night's sleep. The NHS Eatwell guide suggests we drink six to eight glasses of fluid per day; some of this quota can include decaffeinated tea, low-fat milk and sugar-free drinks.

A note on making changes to your diet

Anyone with special dietary requirements (such as those with coeliac disease or type 1 or type 2 diabetes) should always talk things through with their doctor before changing their eating regime.

Exercise

Keeping yourself fit is essential as you transition towards menopause, and is crucial for your long-term health. Regular physical activity at this stage in life helps to:

- Build muscle.
- Strengthen bones.
- Control stress and anxiety levels.
- Boost mood and mindset.
- Lower blood pressure.
- Increase metabolism.
- Maintain a healthy weight.
- Promote social interaction.

I recommend a minimum of 25 minutes of exercise, five days a week. Ideally, this should comprise a combination of resistance training – with free weights or fixed weights – and weight-bearing and cardiovascular workouts such as running, walking, swimming or dancing. This regime can also be complemented with regular stretching, strengthening and breathing exercises, such as those practised in yoga or pilates. Now I know it can feel difficult to fit exercise into a busy life, but remember that every little helps. I like to pepper my day with exercise 'snacks', and have listed a few ideas over the page to get you started.

Osteoporosis is an incredibly debilitating condition, and can severely affect your quality of life. I know patients in their sixties and seventies suffering with poor bone strength who struggle to walk short distances, who are unable to carry their grandchildren, and who can't even lift themselves up off the toilet. So that's why it's massively important to consider your long-term health and put measures into place before it's too late. You will also find some exercise-related resources in the Resources section from page 217.

Exercise 'snacks'

- Get off the bus or train a couple of stops early and finish your journey with a brisk walk.
- Jump off the sofa and try doing a few squats while you're watching TV.
- Exercise your pelvic floor muscles with a quick 'squeeze and lift' movement whenever you stop at traffic lights.
- Clench and release your buttock muscles while you wait in line for your morning coffee.
- Try a few push-ups off the kitchen counter while you're waiting for the kettle to boil.
- Use time that you're catching up with friends and family on the phone as an excuse to get out walking, or ask a colleague to switch a regular meeting into a 'walk and talk' session instead.

Histamine intolerance

Histamine is a compound that is released by cells all over our body and works on our nerves to produce itching. Histamine intolerance happens when our immune system mistakenly believes that a harmless substance is actually harmful to the body.

Histamine intolerance is an issue that's only recently entered the menopause arena, and it's really piqued my interest. So what is it, exactly? Well, oestrogen is an immune modulator – a substance that helps support the immune system to fight disease and infection – and, if it goes into decline, your immune system thinks it's under attack and over-produces histamine.

Symptoms of histamine intolerance

- **Bloating**
- **Headaches**
- **Nausea**
- **Rashes and itchiness**

Histamine intolerance means your system is unable to sufficiently break down the excessive histamine. Added to this, it is believed (but under-researched) that levels of the digestive enzyme diamine oxidase (DAO) are reduced during perimenopause, which further exacerbates histamine intolerance so that some women suddenly find themselves unable to tolerate certain foods. The worst culprits are foods that contain high levels of 'biogenic amines' (amino acids that are released when fermentation takes place) such as processed meat, canned fish, fermented vegetables, mature cheese and red wine.

Conversely (and confusingly) some women who are given oestrogen HRT also experience a surge in histamine levels – sparking similar reactions to those detailed on the previous page – which, again, we think occurs as the body tries to defend itself.

Diagnosis of histamine intolerance

Histamine intolerance is not a well-known condition and currently diagnosis is simply through the discussion of symptoms with your doctor. However, midlife women – as well as their doctors – will often mistake symptoms of histamine intolerance for an allergic reaction, pure and simple, when in fact the underlying trigger is more likely to be hormonal. You can measure DAO activity in the blood serum histamine level, but this is not currently available on the NHS.

Treatment of histamine intolerance

People who've just started HRT can be justifiably alarmed to experience these symptoms – some even consider stopping their treatment – but I would urge you to hang fire and talk to your doctor as there are a number of treatment options:

- **Reduction of histamine-rich foods in your diet**, which would take 14 days to deduce a difference. (I am not endorsing an elimination diet here, but be mindful of what foods cause a reaction for you.)

- **Low-dose antihistamines** such as cetirizine or loratadine – commonly used as hay fever remedies – can be taken to counteract symptoms (I often recommend a three-month course of 10 milligrams per night), after consultation with a medical professional.
- **The anti-nausea drug stemetil** can also be beneficial after consultation with a medical professional.
- **Changing your dose of systemic HRT** (or moving to topical vaginal HRT only), but think carefully about the wider benefits that you may risk losing, too.

COMPLEMENTARY & ALTERNATIVE THERAPIES

The perimenopause is a perfectly normal transition in life, when your periods stop and your oestrogen and progesterone levels are declining. Many women take an holistic approach to their health during this phase, using alternative therapies on a stand-alone basis or to complement more conventional treatments. They might also reassess their lifestyle, perhaps cutting down on alcohol, taking more exercise and trying to reduce their stress at work.

As an NHS doctor, I have no qualms chatting about alternative remedies in my clinic – I use a few of them myself – but I'm also mindful that there can be a lack of evidence-based research surrounding them. While I'm happy to help navigate patients around the various options – and signpost them to relevant resources – it's ultimately up to them to find out what suits them best, from mindfulness and meditation to reiki and reflexology (see Resources from page 217).

Being an NHS doctor, I can't endorse complementary therapies to my patients. However, I'm happy enough to be told anecdotally that something is easing their menopause symptoms. The following therapies are most often cited in my surgery.

Acupuncture

Acupuncture – the ancient Chinese practice of inserting thin needles into the body – is reported to lower hot flushes and night sweats. See Resources from page 217 to help you find an accredited therapist.

Herbal treatments

Herbal therapy has grown in popularity over the years, and I've known many women who swear by Korean ginseng, red clover, black cohosh or St John's wort to manage their perimenopausal symptoms. However, it's very important that these therapies are taken with care, as they can interfere with other medicines. Women on tamoxifen (a post breast cancer hormone-suppressing treatment) should avoid St John's wort, for example, and, in some cases, black cohosh has been known to cause liver toxicity. To ensure that you're taking a regulated product, check for the Herbal Register Stamp before you purchase. See Resources from page 217 to help you find an accredited practitioner.

Cognitive behavioural therapy

Cognitive behavioural therapy (CBT), according to the NHS, is 'a talking therapy that can help you manage your problems by changing the way you think and behave'. Indeed, the National Institute for Health and Care Excellence (NICE) now recommends it as a therapeutic option to alleviate feelings of stress, anxiety and low mood that can be experienced during perimenopause, menopause and post-menopause. Some patients greatly benefit from it – either via self-help, or by working with a qualified specialist – but others find it pretty fruitless and ineffective; it can be a tricky concept to grasp, and needs a lot of practice and application. Like many elements of menopause treatment, there's no one template that suits everybody; it really is a case of 'each to their own'.

Cognitive and behavioural strategies such as breathing exercises and managing your thought processes are known to help with hot flushes. This common menopausal symptom can be quite embarrassing and uncomfortable for those who experience it, especially when it happens in public. Paced, controlled breathing, in which you relax your body and breathe from your stomach, can be really beneficial, as can learning how to manage your feelings when that tell-tale flush engulfs you.

CBT can also help with sleep issues. Many perimenopausal women suffer with insomnia – often worsened by night sweats – yet this can often be controlled by changing your bedtime behaviour and restructuring your thought patterns. This might involve deploying some relaxation techniques, or removing certain sleep distractions (including putting that pesky mobile phone in a drawer!).

CBT is widely available on the NHS everywhere, especially in light of the pandemic, as part of the government's Every Mind Matters initiative. Alternatively, you can try CBT on a self-help basis, without being referred by your doctor (see Resources from page 217).

If you are on HRT, you should always tell your doctor if you're taking complementary medicines.

Acceptance & commitment therapy

An increasing number of my patients with menopausal symptoms, particularly hot flushes, are practising acceptance and commitment therapy (ACT), although it's widely available on the NHS. At its core, ACT is a mindfulness-based therapy that encourages you to accept your situation as it is, rather than fighting against it, which may sometimes mean learning to take the rough with the smooth. An ACT therapist will also help you to commit to tackling issues head on, rather than avoiding them, and will also teach you to manage your negative thoughts.

HORMONE REPLACEMENT THERAPY

There are myriad ways to tackle perimenopause and menopause and minimize symptoms, and as a healthcare professional it's my job to look at each person, assess their situation and connect the dots. A patient can have hormonal treatments and/or non-hormonal treatments – all have pros and cons, and risks and benefits – and during the first consultation, we will work closely together to ascertain how best to manage symptoms. Going down the non-hormonal route is often my first starting point, which generally involves embracing an holistic approach to diet, exercise and lifestyle (see pages 106–12). That being said, many of my patients have already tried those lifestyle changes before they come to see me.

For those individuals whose symptoms are not improved by this non-hormonal course of action, and whose quality of life is still suffering as a result, hormone replacement therapy (HRT) can be a fantastically beneficial treatment. HRT doesn't suit everyone – and I never pressure a patient to take it – but as a doctor who's successfully issued it to hundreds of patients, I can bear witness to its transformative effects.

How HRT works

HRT is simply a supplementation of the hormones that are lacking in a woman's body as she transitions towards the menopause. It consists of two hormones that I've mentioned often in this book – oestrogen and progesterone – and, in some cases, can incorporate a third hormone, testosterone. Women (and those assigned female at birth) who have a uterus will ordinarily use a combination of oestrogen *and* progesterone – this is to prevent the thickening of the endometrial lining of the uterus, which can be caused by oestrogen-only treatment. But those who've had a hysterectomy will usually take oestrogen by itself.

Hormone replacement therapy is designed to relieve a whole host of troublesome perimenopausal symptoms including palpitations, insomnia and depression (see pages 67–70 for the full list). Studies suggest it may have long-term benefits, too, including a reduced risk of osteoporosis, dementia, type 2 diabetes, depression and cardiovascular disease.

HRT is available on prescription in a variety of preparations and combinations and, depending on the woman's individual needs, some types can be adjusted and fine-tuned on a day-to-day basis. This is ideal for women who have cyclical symptoms which vary in intensity. HRT is also available as 'systemic HRT' – tablets, patches or gels that treat symptoms throughout the body; or 'topical HRT' – creams, gels and pessaries that only treat symptoms in the genitals.

By seeking help and guidance from your doctor – and by allowing yourself time and patience to discover your best 'fit' – you can benefit from a bespoke HRT regime to control your hormones and ease your symptoms. What's not to love?

Using HRT

HRT is usually offered to three groups of patients:

- **Those showing classic perimenopausal symptoms** who wish to relieve the symptoms.
- **Those who experience premature ovarian insufficiency** (POI), surgical menopause or chemical menopause (see page 63).
- **Those with perimenopausal symptoms** who want to protect themselves against osteoporosis and other conditions such as heart disease and vascular dementia.

I choose not to apply an upper or lower age limit when I prescribe HRT, simply because the needs of my patients are paramount. They may be 43, or 53, or 63, but if they're sitting in my surgery, struggling with a litany of tell-tale symptoms, I'll gladly discuss the pros and cons of HRT.

In my experience, women wait until their symptoms get really bad, about four years, before going on systemic HRT. It doesn't have to be this way! Don't wait until your symptoms get severe before plucking up the courage to talk about HRT with your doctor.

Unlike other medications, HRT is not given as a course of treatment and, if it aids a woman's health and wellbeing, there's no reason why it can't be taken indefinitely (essentially for the rest of a woman's life). HRT does not delay menopause – that's a question I'm often asked – but simply controls symptoms while they are present.

Minor side effects are common in the first few weeks of HRT treatment – such as nausea, leg cramps and breast tenderness – so I often advise my patients to persevere during these early stages. Once everything has settled down, any side effects can be minimized by adjusting HRT types and doses.

Over 1/3 of women who visited their doctor with perimenopausal symptoms were offered antidepressants

HRT treatment formats

There are a few different ways to take HRT:

- **Oral tablets and capsules** are usually taken daily so they are easy to remember. Oestrogen tablets are associated with a slightly higher risk of clots than patches or gels, because they are processed by the liver. They can also lower libido and may not be suitable if you are obese or have certain health conditions. They

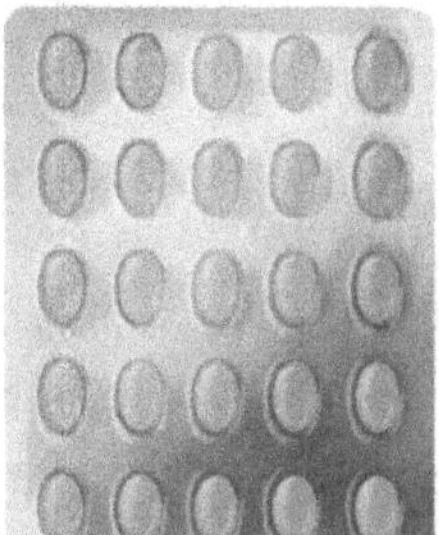

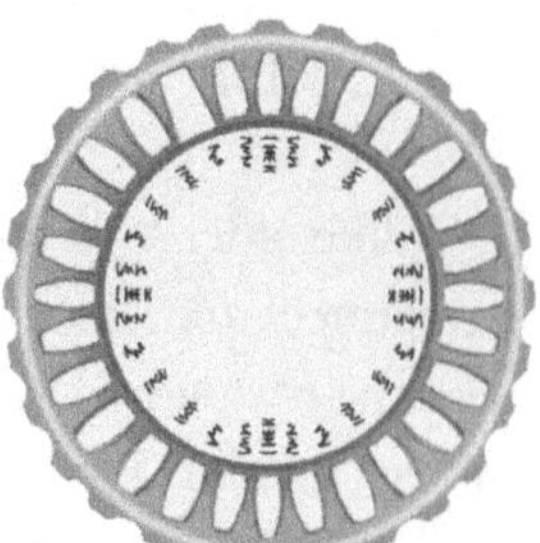

can be less reliable in terms of absorption if you have an upset stomach.

- **Skin patches** are stuck onto the skin and changed once or twice a week. These give a constant dose so can be good if you suffer from migraines. You can also use multiple patches if you need a higher dose. The adhesive used can leave a sticky residue, but that can be easily removed with baby oil.

- **Skin gels and sprays** are usually rubbed over your arms or legs. They make it easy to control the dose so your doctor can tailor a very specific dose according to your

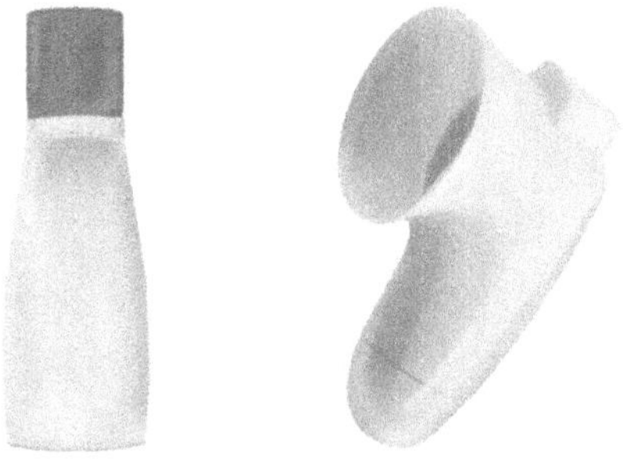

requirements or advise you to use them in conjunction with a patch. They can ease PMS symptoms if you still have periods, and the dose can be increased for the days before your period if necessary.

- **Implants** are inserted by a healthcare practitioner and can be useful for women who do not absorb oestrogen well. However, they can lead to fluctuating hormone levels and doses are less flexible than in other formats.

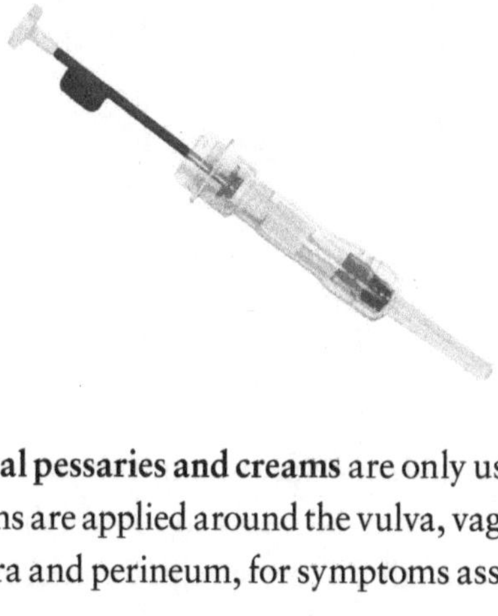

- **Vaginal pessaries and creams** are only used topically. Creams are applied around the vulva, vagina, bladder, urethra and perineum, for symptoms associated with

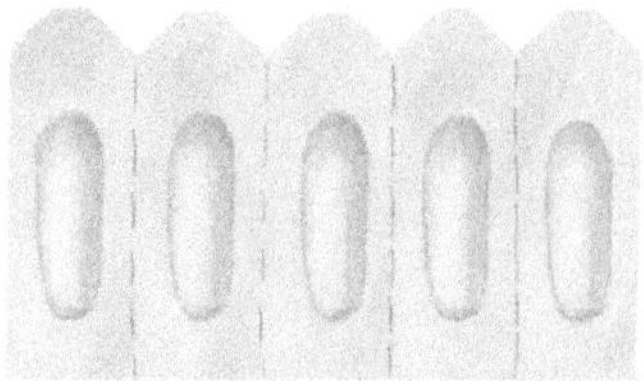

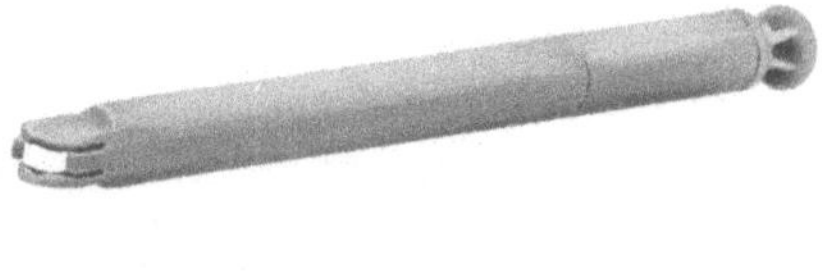

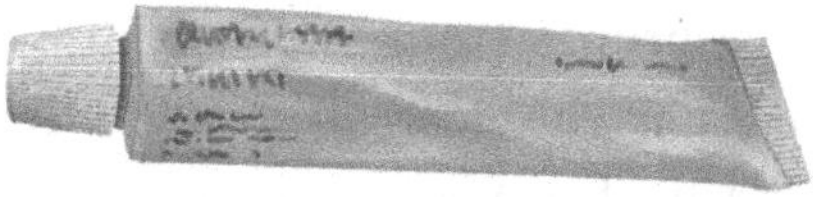

the lowering of oestrogen levels in the body, while pessaries are inserted into the vagina.

HRT treatment types

The best HRT treatment for you depends on your personal circumstances. In general, they can be classified as one of the following:

- **Combined HRT** contains both oestrogen (which relieves menopausal symptoms) and progesterone (which reduces the risk of oestrogen causing abnormal changes to the lining of the womb). If you still have periods (whether monthly or irregularly), you would usually take the oestrogen element continually and the progesterone element for two weeks in every four. If you are post-menopausal, you would take the treatment continually.
- **Oestrogen-only HRT** is suitable if you have had a hysterectomy. People who have had a hysterectomy do not usually need to include progesterone in their HRT as there is no risk of their oestrogen treatment causing abnormal changes to the lining of the uterus (since it has been removed). However, if you've had a hysterectomy as a result of severe endometriosis, then your doctor might want to

include a progesterone supplementation in case there are any endometrial cells left in the pelvis. Similarly, if a hysterectomy didn't include removal of the cervix, then in some cases women might also need progesterone as part of their HRT to prevent any remaining endometrial cells from thickening abnormally. Oestrogen-only HRT can also be taken by those who have not had a hysterectomy if taken alongside a progesterone-only HRT. This can work well for women who find they have unwanted side effects from certain oestrogens or progesterones.

- **Topical vaginal oestrogen** suitable for women who suffer the effects of vaginal atrophy (see page 73). As it is topical, it does not carry the associated risks of other forms of HRT and is therefore suitable for women who have, or have had, oestrogen-receptor positive breast cancer. Topical vaginal oestrogen does not relieve systemic menopausal symptoms.

Body identical HRT

Due to medical and scientific advances, there's a growing list of HRT preparations. The latest, newer-generation treatments are particularly brilliant; they're known as body identical, which means they mimic the chemical shape and structure of our own natural hormones. They are plant-based, and I find myself recommending them, rather than the older-generation, synthetic types of HRT, more frequently. The transdermal body-identical oestrogens – gels, sprays and patches – are perceived as particularly safe options since they're absorbed through the skin rather than being processed by the liver. Body-identical progesterones are also derived from plant-based ingredients, and studies have shown they have fewer risks and side effects than their synthetic counterparts (see page 162). Weighing things up with a medical practitioner will help you decide if the body-identical route is best for you.

Beware compound bio-identical hormones

You may come across references to 'compound bio-identical' hormones, but they should *not* be confused with 'body-identical' hormones. These are in fact unregulated medicines, often marketed as 'natural', that are prescribed privately by specialist clinicians. Neither NICE nor the British Menopause Society (BMS) believe these 'bio-identical' products have enough robust data to demonstrate their safety and efficacy (please check out the BMS website if you'd like to read more).

Cyclical combined HRT

✓ Suitable for women with a uterus, who have perimenopausal symptoms and still bleed

✓ In a typical cycle, combined oestrogen and progestogen tablets are taken for two weeks in every four and oestrogen-only tablets are taken for two weeks in four

PRODUCT NAME	OESTROGEN TYPE + PROGESTOGEN TYPE	SYNTHETIC (S) OR BODY-IDENTICAL (B)?	DELIVERY	NOTES
Elleste Duet	estradiol + norethisterone acetate	S	oral tablets	• Taken daily so easy to remember • Slight increase in risk of clots • Less reliable absorption than transdermal forms • May not be suitable if you are obese or have type 2 diabetes • First line oral treatment option for most healthcare practitioners
Femoston	estradiol hemihydrate + dydrogesterone	S	oral tablets	• Taken daily so easy to remember • Slight increase in risk of clots • Less reliable absorption than transdermal forms

PRODUCT NAME	OESTROGEN TYPE + PROGESTOGEN TYPE	SYNTHETIC (S) OR BODY-IDENTICAL (B)?	DELIVERY	NOTES
				• May not be suitable if you are obese or have type 2 diabetes • Offered as an alternative if the norethisterone progestogen in Elleste Duet causes side effects, such as erratic bleeding patterns, acne or dizziness
Prempak C	conjugated oestrogens + norgestrel	S	oral tablets	• Taken daily so easy to remember • Slight increase in risk of clots • Less reliable absorption than transdermal forms • May not be suitable if you are obese or have type 2 diabetes • Made from mare's urine, which can deter patients
Evorel Sequi	estradiol hemihydrate + norethisterone acetate	B	transdermal patches	• Adheres to the thigh or buttock and can be worn in the bath, shower or while swimming

continues overleaf

PRODUCT NAME	OESTROGEN TYPE + PROGESTOGEN TYPE	SYNTHETIC (S) OR BODY-IDENTICAL (B)?	DELIVERY	NOTES
				• Offers a constant dose of oestrogen • First line transdermal option for most healthcare practitioners
FemSeven Sequi	estradiol + levonorgestrel	B	transdermal patches	• Adheres to the thigh or buttock and can be worn in the bath, shower or while swimming • Offers a constant dose of oestrogen • Can be used as an alternative if patients have skin allergies, poor absorption or poor adhesion with other patches
Personalized bespoke option	oestrogen of choice + progesterone of choice (most commonly Utrogestan capsules taken cyclically or the Mirena™ IUS coil)	depends on formats chosen	depends on formats chosen	• Can be used if you experience side effects (such as bleeding problems) from the progesterone types used in other combined treatments

* Always consult your own doctor before starting any new treatment.

Continuous combined HRT

- ✓ Suitable for women with a uterus, who have not had a period for more than 12 months
- ✓ The combined oestrogen and progestogen tablets are taken continually

PRODUCT NAME	OESTROGEN TYPE + PROGESTOGEN TYPE	SYNTHETIC (S) OR BODY-IDENTICAL (B)?	DELIVERY	NOTES
Kliovance	estradiol + norethisterone acetate	S	oral tablets	• Taken daily so easy to remember • Slight increase in risk of clots • Less reliable absorption than transdermal forms • May not be suitable if you are obese or have type 2 diabetes • First line oral treatment option for continuous HRT
Femoston Conti	estradiol hemihydrate + dydrogesterone	S	oral tablets	• Taken daily so easy to remember • Slight increase in risk of clots • Less reliable absorption than transdermal forms • May not be suitable if you are obese or have type 2 diabetes

continues overleaf

PRODUCT NAME	OESTROGEN TYPE + PROGESTOGEN TYPE	SYNTHETIC (S) OR BODY-IDENTICAL (B)?	DELIVERY	NOTES
				• An alternative if there are side effects (bloating or tender breast tissue) with other progestogens
Premique low dose	conjugated oestrogens + medroxy-progesterone acetate	S	oral tablets	• Taken daily so easy to remember • Slight increase in risk of clots • Less reliable absorption than transdermal forms • May not be suitable if you are obese or have type 2 diabetes • Usually offered if you have reacted well to cyclical equine oestrogen previously • Made from mare's urine, which can deter patients
Indivina	estradiol + medroxy-progesterone	S	oral tablets	• Taken daily so easy to remember • Slight increase in risk of clots • Less reliable absorption than transdermal forms

PRODUCT NAME	OESTROGEN TYPE + PROGESTOGEN TYPE	SYNTHETIC (S) OR BODY-IDENTICAL (B)?	DELIVERY	NOTES
				• May not be suitable if you are obese or have type 2 diabetes • Offered if you have had bleeding on other forms of continuous combined HRT and uterine pathology has been ruled out (including polyps, fibroids, thickening of endometrial lining)
Angeliq	estradiol + drospirenone	S	oral tablets	• Taken daily so easy to remember • Slight increase in risk of clots • Less reliable absorption than transdermal forms • May not be suitable if you are obese or have type 2 diabetes • Can be used as an alternative if there are side effects with other progestogen types (such as bloating, acne or tender breast tissue)

continues overleaf

PRODUCT NAME	OESTROGEN TYPE + PROGESTOGEN TYPE	SYNTHETIC (S) OR BODY-IDENTICAL (B)?	DELIVERY	NOTES
Tibolone	tibolone (a synthetic molecule with oestrogen, progestogen and androgenic properties)	S	oral tablets	• Taken daily so easy to remember • Slight increase in risk of clots • Less reliable absorption than transdermal forms • May not be suitable if you are obese or have type 2 diabetes • The androgenic properties have been found to improve low libido in some studies • Can also be considered post hysterectomy and/or bilateral salpingo oophorectomy (BSO)
Bijuve	estradiol hemihydrate + progesterone	S + B	oral capsules	• Taken daily so easy to remember • Less reliable absorption than transdermal forms

PRODUCT NAME	OESTROGEN TYPE + PROGESTOGEN TYPE	SYNTHETIC (S) OR BODY-IDENTICAL (B)?	DELIVERY	NOTES
				• Unlike other oral tablets, this is more suitable for women who have clot and migraine history because it contains body-identical micronized progesterone • The risk of breast cancer is lower in younger women compared with oral synthetic continuous combined HRT
Evorel Conti	estradiol hemihydrate + norethisterone acetate	B + S	transdermal patches	• Adheres to the thigh or buttock and can be worn in the bath, shower or while swimming • Offers a constant dose of oestrogen • First line treatment for transdermal continual HRT • Patches applied twice a week

continues overleaf

PRODUCT NAME	OESTROGEN TYPE + PROGESTOGEN TYPE	SYNTHETIC (S) OR BODY-IDENTICAL (B)?	DELIVERY	NOTES
FemSeven Conti	estradiol hemihydrate + levonorgetrel	B + S	transdermal patches	• Adheres to the thigh or buttock and can be worn in the bath, shower or while swimming • Offers a constant dose of oestrogen • Can be used as an alternative if patients have skin allergies, poor absorption or poor adhesion with other patches
Personalized bespoke option	Oestrogen of choice + progesterone of choice (most commonly Utrogestan capsules taken continually or the Mirena™ IUS coil)	depends on formats chosen	depends on formats chosen	• Can be used if you experience side effects (such as bleeding problems) from the progesterone types used in other combined treatments

* Always consult your own doctor before starting any new treatment.

In my clinical experience, there is NO individual who cannot have treatment in some form to help relieve menopausal symptoms, even those who have (or have had) cancer.

Oestrogen-only HRT

✓ Suitable for women who've had a hysterectomy (so have no uterus)

✓ Suitable for women who still have a uterus but want to take progestogens separately

PRODUCT NAME	OESTROGEN TYPE	SYNTHETIC (S) OR BODY-IDENTICAL (B)?	DELIVERY	NOTES
Elleste Solo	estradiol	S	oral tablets	• Taken daily so easy to remember • Slight increase in risk of clots • Can lower libido • Less reliable absorption than transdermal forms • May not be suitable if you are obese or have type 2 diabetes
Premarin	conjugated oestrogens	S	oral tablets	• Taken daily so easy to remember • Slight increase in risk of clots • Can lower libido • Less reliable absorption than transdermal forms • May not be suitable if you are obese or have type 2 diabetes • Made from mare's urine, which can deter patients

PRODUCT NAME	OESTROGEN TYPE	SYNTHETIC (S) OR BODY-IDENTICAL (B)?	DELIVERY	NOTES
Evorel	estradiol	B	transdermal patches	• Adheres to the thigh or buttock and can be worn in the bath, shower and while swimming • Offers a constant dose of oestrogen • Change twice weekly
Elleste Solo MX	estradiol hemihydrate	B	transdermal patches	• Adheres to the thigh or buttock and can be worn in the bath, shower and while swimming • Offers a constant dose of oestrogen • Can be used as an alternative if other patches cause skin allergies, or have poor absorption/adhesion • Change twice weekly
Estradot	estradiol hemihydrate	B	transdermal patches	• Adheres to the thigh or buttock and can be worn in the bath, shower and while swimming • Offers a constant dose of oestrogen • Available in smaller-sized patches with a higher concentration of active ingredients, so more suitable for higher doses and petite women • Change twice weekly

continues overleaf

PRODUCT NAME	OESTROGEN TYPE	SYNTHETIC (S) OR BODY-IDENTICAL (B)?	DELIVERY	NOTES
FemSeven Mono	estrodiol hemihydrate	B	transdermal patch	• Adheres to the thigh or buttock and can be worn in the bath, shower and while swimming • Offers a constant dose of oestrogen • Available in smaller-sized patches with a higher concentration of active ingredients, so more suitable for higher doses and petite women • Change every 7 days
Estraderm MX	estradiol	B	transdermal patches	• Adheres to the thigh or buttock and can be worn in the bath, shower and while swimming • Offers a constant dose of oestrogen • Change twice weekly
Progynova TS	estradiol	B	transdermal patches	• Adheres to the thigh or buttock and can be worn in the bath, shower and while swimming • Offers a constant dose of oestrogen • Can be cut into halves or quarters for dose adjustments • Change every 7 days

PRODUCT NAME	OESTROGEN TYPE	SYNTHETIC(S) OR BODY-IDENTICAL (B)?	DELIVERY	NOTES
Sandrena	estradiol hemihydrate	B	transdermal gel (sachet)	• Very easy to use • Simple to regulate dosage if symptoms are cyclical • Can be used as an alternative if patches cause skin allergies • Individual sachets are less environmentally friendly than other options
Oestrogel	estradiol hemihydrate	B	transdermal gel (bottle)	• Very easy-to-use and a highly popular option with patients • The 100ml bottle can be taken in hand luggage • Simple to regulate dosage if symptoms are cyclical • Can be used as an alternative if patches cause skin allergies • Plastic bottle can be recycled • Can be subject to shortages

continues overleaf

PRODUCT NAME	OESTROGEN TYPE	SYNTHETIC (S) OR BODY-IDENTICAL (B)?	DELIVERY	NOTES
Lenzetto	estradiol hemihydrate	B	transdermal spray	• A very light, easily absorbed preparation that is sprayed onto skin • Simple to regulate dosage if symptoms are cyclical • Can be used as an alternative if patches cause skin allergies • Currently more expensive in comparison to other formulas so some doctors may be reluctant to prescribe

* Always consult your own doctor before starting any new treatment.

Topical vaginal oestrogen

- ✓ Suitable for women with symptoms relating to genito-urinary syndrome of the menopause, which includes dryness, burning, itching, painful sex and recurrent UTIs
- ✓ Vaginal oestrogen does not ease other perimenopause/menopause-related systemic symptoms

PRODUCT NAME	OESTROGEN TYPE	DELIVERY	NOTES
Vagifem	estradiol	vaginal pessary	• Self-administered in a single-use applicator • A number of treatments are usually required • Use one pessary every night for 2 weeks and then reduce to 2–5 times a week, settling on the frequency that relieves your symptoms • Safe for women with breast cancer on Tamoxifen
Vagirux	estradiol	vaginal pessary	• Self-administered with a reusable applicator • A number of treatments are usually required • Use one pessary every night for 2 weeks and then reduce to 2–5 times a week, settling on the frequency that relieves your symptoms • Safe for women with breast cancer on Tamoxifen • Suitable for women with a past history of breast cancer, who are not currently on AI or Tamoxifen, if Estring is not tolerated

continues overleaf

PRODUCT NAME	OESTROGEN TYPE	DELIVERY	NOTES
Imvaggis	estriol	vaginal pessary	• Very low dose format • Highly lubricated and easy to insert • Self-administered with a reusable applicator • A number of treatments are usually required • Use one pessary every night for 2 weeks and then reduce to twice a week, although guidelines allow up to 5 times a week at your doctor's discretion
Gina	estradiol	vaginal pessary	• Available over the counter in the UK, for women over the age of 50 who have not had a period for at least one year and who have vaginal menopausal symptoms • Self-administered with a reusable applicator • A number of treatments are usually required • Use one pessary every night for 2 weeks and then reduce to 2–5 times a week, settling on the frequency that relieves your symptoms
Gynest/ Estriol/ 0.01%	estriol	vaginal cream	• Self-administered with a reusable applicator • Some find a cream more comfortable to insert than a pessary • A number of treatments are usually required • Use one dose every night for 2 weeks and then reduce to twice a week, although guidelines allow up to 5 times a week at your doctor's discretion

PRODUCT NAME	OESTROGEN TYPE	DELIVERY	NOTES
Ovestin	estriol	vaginal cream	• Self-administered with a finger or a reusable applicator • Can be applied externally to just the vulva as well as internally into the vagina • A number of treatments are usually required • Use one dose every night for 2 weeks and then reduce to twice a week, although guidelines allow up to 5 times a week at your doctor's discretion
Generic creams	estradiol	vaginal cream	• A number of generic creams are available on prescription • Self-administered with a finger or an applicator • These can be oily so are not condom-friendly and can be messy • They can contain peanut oil unsuitable for those with an allergy • The length of time that effects last varies according to the brand
Estring	estradiol	vaginal ring	• This flexible ring is inserted in a similar manner to a tampon • Can be fitted yourself or by your doctor • Effects last for 3 months per insertion, so it is useful and effective for women who can't manage daily use themselves • You can leave it in to have sex or it can be removed if needed • Good alternative if you find yourself using Vagifem or Vagirux at the maximum established dose of five times a week

continues overleaf

PRODUCT NAME	OESTROGEN TYPE	DELIVERY	NOTES
			• Safe for use by women who have had, or currently have, breast cancer on Aromatase Inhibitors (AI, such as Anastrozole or Exemestane), because it provides a constant slow release of topical oestrogen, rather than loading 2 or 3 times weekly • First line for women with a past history of breast cancer, who are not currently on AI or Tamoxifen
Blissel	estriol	vaginal gel	• Self-administered with a reusable applicator • Highly hydrating and non-greasy • A number of treatments are usually required • Use one dose every night for 2–3 weeks and then reduce to twice a week, although guidelines allow up to 5 times a week at your doctor's discretion • Slightly more expensive than other products so doctors may be reluctant to prescribe
Intrarosa DHEA/ Parastone DHEA	DHEA (an androgen that converts into an oestrogen when in the body)	topical pessary	• Self-administered with a reusable applicator • Inserted into the vagina once daily at bedtime • Highly hydrating and non-greasy • A number of treatments are usually required • Safe to use for patients who have had, or currently have, breast cancer and are on aromatase inhibitors (such as Anastrozole or Exemestane)

* Always consult your own doctor before starting any new treatment.

Progestogens & progesterones

- ✓ Suitable for women with a uterus who do not want to take a combined HRT treatment
- ✓ Progesterone on its own does not relieve perimenopausal/menopausal symptoms but is used in combination with an oestrogen-only treatment to reduce the risks of oestrogen-only treatment

PRODUCT NAME	PROGESTERONE/ PROGESTOGEN TYPE	SYNTHETIC (S) OR BODY-IDENTICAL (B)?	DELIVERY	NOTES
Utrogestan	progesterone	B	oral capsules	• Cyclical regime for women who are menstruating: 200mg at bedtime for 2 weeks out of 4 • Continuous combined regime for women whose periods have stopped for a year: 100mg at bedtime, daily • The oral capsules can also be taken vaginally (at half the oral dose, at the discretion of your menopause specialist) to avoid side effects, such as bloating, acne, dizziness, low mood or other progesterone intolerance symptoms

continues overleaf

PRODUCT NAME	PROGESTERONE/ PROGESTOGEN TYPE	SYNTHETIC (S) OR BODY-IDENTICAL (B)?	DELIVERY	NOTES
Provera	medroxy-progesterone acetate	S	oral tablets	• Cyclical regime for women who are menstruating: 10mg at bedtime for 2 weeks out of 4 • Continuous combined regime for women whose periods have stopped for a year: 2.5–5mg at bedtime, daily
Norethis-terone	Norethisterone	S	Oral tablet	• Cyclical regime for women who are menstruating: 5mg at bedtime for 12 days a month. • Continuous combined regime for women whose whose periods have stopped for a year: 5mg at bedtime on a continuous basis.
Noriday	norothisterone	S	oral tablets	• Continuous combined regime for women whose periods have stopped for a year: 3 x 350mg tablets a day – this will provide 1.05mg of norothisterone • This is an off-license use of a protesterone-only contraceptive pill.

PRODUCT NAME	PROGESTERONE/ PROGESTOGEN TYPE	SYNTHETIC(S) OR BODY-IDENTICAL(B)?	DELIVERY	NOTES
Slynd®	Drospirenone	S	oral tablets	• Continuous combined regime for women whose periods have stopped for a year: 4mg daily on a continuous basis, omitting the 4 hormone-free pills in the packet • This is an off licence use of a progesterone-only contraceptive pill that can be considered in a continuous combined HRT regime for women who experience prostogenic side effects (such as acne, low mood, hair thinning etc) with other preparations
Intrauterine system (Mirena™ IUS coil)	levonorgestrel	S	coil inserted into uterus by clinician	• Also acts as a contraceptive • Can stop heavy periods • Insertion can be painful and initially cause erratic bleeding • Each coil lasts for 5 years for HRT use, after which it can be renewed

continues overleaf

PRODUCT NAME	PROGESTERONE/ PROGESTOGEN TYPE	SYNTHETIC(S) OR BODY-IDENTICAL (B)?	DELIVERY	NOTES
Cyclogest/ Lutigest	progesterone	B	vaginal pessary	• Commonly used as part of fertility treatments • If they are experiencing progesterone intolerance, some women prefer to use these (off licence at the discretion of your menopause specialist)

* Always consult your own doctor before starting any new treatment.

A note about stopping sequential/ cyclical HRT regimes

Some patients ask me when they should stop taking progesterone cyclically, and transfer over to a continuous regime. If you're on a combined sequential/cyclical regime that contains oestrogen and the progesterone-only mini-pill, your fertility is suppressed, so you won't have periods and therefore won't be able to gauge when you're medically menopausal. So, if you're under the age of 45 your doctor will need to stop your HRT regime for four weeks before giving you two blood tests, six weeks apart, to check your levels of oestrogen and follicle stimulating hormone (FSH) in order to establish whether you're menopausal and need to change your regime. But if you're above the age of 45, your doctor won't deem it necessary to perform a blood test and will just switch you over to continuous HRT.

If you're on a combined sequential/cyclical regime that consists of an oestrogen-only product taken alongside progesterone, your fertility is not suppressed, so you will still be menstruating. However, once your periods reach a natural cessation – and you don't experience a bleed for 12 months – you'll be deemed menopausal and will be switched over to continuous HRT.

A note about the progesterone coil & progesterone-only pill

If you have a progesterone coil or are taking the progesterone-only pill and are not having periods, and are wondering 'Am I in the menopause?', you can seek help from your doctor. If you're over the age of 45, you'll probably not need a blood test; your doctor will diagnose you by your symptoms alone. Women under the age of 45 can be given the FSH test, and your doctor may also check for issues such as anaemia and thyroid function, liver and kidney function.

'Off licence' refers to using medication in a way that's not typically recommended by the manufacturer. It does not make the suggested usage clinically unsafe as it's commonly practised under the guidance of doctors and other medical professionals.

Testosterone

There's been a lot of debate around testosterone. Contrary to popular belief, testosterone is not just a male preserve; women actually need it, too. It contributes to libido, orgasm and sexual arousal, and plays a vital role in maintaining urogenital health, muscle and bone strength, skin collagen levels and cognitive function. It's a hormone that has many roles to play and, whenever we talk about HRT treatment for menopausal symptoms, it should definitely form part of that conversation.

If your doctor is treating you for low sexual desire with testosterone therapy, it is important that urogenital tissues are adequately treated with vaginal oestrogen (see page 78) to avoid painful or uncomfortable sex.

Testosterone can be taken alongside an oestrogen and progesterone HRT regime, and is usually a gel-based treatment that is easily rubbed onto the skin. However, this hormone should only be prescribed by a doctor like myself who is specially trained in testosterone therapy for low sexual desire, once a bio-psychosocial approach has excluded relationship issues, stress, and anti-depressant medications such as SSRIs or SNRIs (see page 174).

As I write, there is no uniformed way of prescribing testosterone in the UK. Other countries, including Australia, willingly prescribe this hormone to women, so why can't we? The Aussies have even produced a female-specific preparation (Androgel/Androfeme, see page 154) so I can only assume that they attach more value to a woman's sex life than the Brits!

While it's possible for a patient to receive testosterone treatment, getting a prescription isn't always straightforward. More often than not, the patient's symptoms alone will tell the story and will allow the clinician to make a sensible diagnosis, but when they request testosterone, they will have to undergo a blood test to measure their base levels of androgens – a group of sex hormones – and to check that there aren't any other underlying and treatable reasons for any deficit.

Testosterone isn't an instant fix – it can take a few months for a person to notice any clinical difference – but, when it does kick in, the effects can be remarkable. Patients of mine have reported a massive increase in their sex drive and their general wellbeing, which is a pretty wonderful outcome for all concerned!

However, if a patient hasn't noticed any difference after six months, the British Menopause Society (BMS) guidelines suggest that the testosterone treatment should be stopped, and other management avenues should be explored.

As of October 2022, the British Menopause Guidelines state that for all testosterone products, your total testosterone level should be checked before treatment begins. After six weeks of use, an additional test is required to assess effectiveness. Once on an established dose, monitoring continues every 6–12 months to ensure that the levels remain within the female physiological range.

Testosterone treatments

- ✓ Suitable for women with low libido
- ✓ Can also contribute to good urogenital health, and help muscle and bone strength and cognitive function

PRODUCT NAME	DELIVERY	NOTES
Androfeme	transdermal cream	• The only testosterone cream that is currently licensed for use in women in the UK • Can take several months to work • Frequency of use is at the discretion of your menopause specialist • Synthesized from soya so not suitable if you have an allergy
Androgel	transdermal gel	• The only testosterone gel that is currently licensed for use in women in the UK • Can take several months to work • Frequency of use is at the discretion of your menopause specialist • Synthesized from soya so not suitable if you have an allergy
Testogel	transdermal gel	• Licensed for use in men; can be used off licence to provide female physiological testosterone replacement • Available in sachets • Can take several months to work • Frequency of use is at the discretion of your menopause specialist

PRODUCT NAME	DELIVERY	NOTES
Testim	transdermal gel	• Licensed for use in men; can be used off licence to provide female physiological testosterone replacement • Available in a canister • Can take several months to work • Frequency of use is at the discretion of your menopause specialist
Tostran	transdermal gel	• Licensed for use in men; can be used off licence to provide female physiological testosterone replacement • Available in a canister • Can take several months to work • Frequency of use is at the discretion of your menopause specialist

* Always consult your own doctor before starting any new treatment.

THE RISKS OF HORMONE REPLACEMENT THERAPY

There are potential risks for some women taking HRT, as there are with most medical treatments, so it's important to arm yourself with the facts before embarking on treatment. However, I believe that all women can find something suitable for their level of risk and current situation to help their symptoms.

Not every woman is a candidate for HRT when the risks can potentially outweigh the benefits, and as doctors we look at individual symptoms as best we can. If you're considering HRT, you need to discuss your own particular circumstances with your doctor so request a double appointment if you can. Your age, lifestyle, medical history and personal preference will be taken into account.

For the majority of women who are prescribed HRT, I believe the pros considerably outweigh the cons. I, like many of my colleagues, believe that the newer, body-identical HRT products not only effectively manage the symptoms of perimenopause, but can also lessen the risk of conditions such as osteoporosis, vascular dementia and heart disease. Preventative care is the core principle of the NHS, when all is said and done, and I think HRT perfectly fits that purpose. Indeed, since 2019, the guidance from the National Institute for Health and Care Excellence (NICE) is clear that HRT should be recommended as a first-line therapy to perimenopausal women to help symptom control and to aid future health.

There are some risks with HRT and, if you want to find out what's best for you, you need to discuss the pros and cons with your doctor face-to-face and, if possible, arm yourself with evidence-based research (see Resources from page 217).

All I would say, though, is that I've known some individuals who are eligible for HRT but, being fearful of the risks, decide against using it and continue to suffer horrendous perimenopausal symptoms. So my message is: please don't deny yourself HRT without thoroughly exploring the upsides and downsides.

As regards HRT, always ask yourself, 'Do the benefits outweigh the risks?'

IMPORTANT!

We need to stop scaring women about oestrogen, and instead empower them with evidence-based information.

Understanding the risks of breast cancer

The following is a comparison of lifestyle risk factors versus hormone replacement therapy (HRT) treatment and their effect on the estimated difference in breast cancer incidence per 1,000 women aged 50–59 over the next five years:

As a baseline, in the general UK population, approximately 23 women per 1,000 are diagnosed with breast cancer. Current evidence suggests that women on combined HRT may see around four additional cases (27 women per 1,000), the same incidence as those using a combined hormonal contraceptive (the pill). However, those using oestrogen-only HRT may experience four fewer cases. Lifestyle factors also have a notable impact: drinking two or more units of alcohol per day is linked to five extra cases; smoking to an additional three; and being overweight or obese (BMI ≥30) to 24 extra cases. In contrast, regular physical activity – at least 2½ hours of moderate exercise per week – is associated with seven fewer cases.

Please refer to the Women's Health Concern website for the latest information: http://www.womens-health-concern.org.

Breast cancer & HRT

Breast cancer (see pages 191–94) is a life-changing disease that affects millions of women across the globe. Although it is commonly linked to old age those in younger age groups, or those assigned female at birth with breast tissue, can also contract it. In the UK, one in seven women will develop the disease at some point in their life.

In the past, some clinical studies have linked breast cancer with HRT. The infamous Women's Health Institute study in the early 2000s, for example, which received huge coverage in the media, claimed that synthetic, systemic oestrogen – now regarded as one of the 'older' types of HRT – significantly increased the risk of breast cancer and heart disease. This turned out to be a misleading assertion, closer inspection of the study data showed this heightened risk wasn't solely related to oestrogen. There was a slight increase in women developing breast cancer if they used combined synthetic oestrogen *and* synthetic progesterone HRT, but this amounted to just one in every 1,000 women per year.

However, more recent studies – including a paper entitled 'Menopausal hormone therapy formulation and breast cancer risk', published in June 2022 by the American College of Obstetricians and Gynaecologists – have made it clear that breast cancer risks are comparatively lower among individuals using the new-generation, body-identical versions of HRT. On the previous page is a graphic that I find hugely helpful, courtesy of the BMS, showing the breast cancer risks of HRT versus other factors.

The key facts are as follows:

- Women below the age of 50 using HRT comprising transdermal, body-identical oestrogen and micronized progesterone have a lower relative risk of breast cancer, in comparison with the older version of HRT.

- Women below the age of 50 who've had a hysterectomy (and therefore use transdermal, body-identical oestrogen on its own) do not have an increased risk of breast cancer.
- Women over the age of 50 who choose to take HRT for menopausal symptoms will have a slightly higher risk of breast cancer than those who do not take HRT, but remember: the older you are, the higher your risk is anyway.
- There is no increased risk of breast cancer among women who take vaginal oestrogen to relieve menopausal symptoms (even if they have, or have had, breast cancer).
- Thanks to improved breast screening, far fewer women in the UK are dying from breast cancer nowadays. Screening mammograms – together with the urgent cancer referral system – are helping with early detection and better prognosis.

Self examination of the breasts and breast tissue (at all ages), is the best way to pick up early breast changes.

But fears about oestrogen still linger, despite growing evidence that suggests it does not cause breast cancer alone. As clinicians, we *have* to emphasize to our patients that this is the case, and we need to explain that the wider picture is far more multi-layered. Family health history, biological female status, advancing age and possession of breast tissue will naturally increase the risk of developing breast cancer, as might lifestyle choices relating to diet, exercise, smoking and alcohol. Indeed, according to Cancer Research UK, having a BMI above 30 increases your chances of breast cancer by 50 per cent in women over the age of 50. Drinking two or more glasses of wine per night (or exceeding the recommended amount of 14 units of alcohol per week) proves to be riskier than taking the newer, body-identical types of HRT.

That said, by suggesting that breast cancer can often be related to lifestyle, age or genetics, I do not wish to alienate, aggravate or in any way 'blame' sufferers and survivors. I sometimes receive kickback online from individuals who feel my observations are unfair, especially if their own health and wellbeing regime has been exemplary, but – along with many other menopause specialists – I just believe that, in general, the benefits of HRT outweigh any potential risks.

I also appreciate that some individuals feel discriminated against because they're unable to take HRT due to a cancer diagnosis, or because of other illnesses or conditions. I am very conscious of this and, whether it's in my surgery or on social media, I'm happy to recommend alternative medical treatments (see pages 173–74) and complementary and alternative therapies (see pages 117–20) that may benefit those patients.

Blood clots & HRT

Studies show that transdermal oestrogen, unlike synthetic oral oestrogen, does not increase the risk of blood clots, known medically as venous thromboembolism (VTE). Also, compared with synthetic progesterones, micronized progesterone shows a reduced risk of clots when used in combination with oestrogen. This means that patients who have migraines, who are overweight, who have a family history of clots (or have had a clot in the past that has been treated) can be considered for body-identical HRT, subject to the risks and benefits being weighed up for each individual patient.

Like all sex hormones, oestrogen is derived from cholesterol, so patients who already have high cholesterol levels or who have underlying heart disease need to be careful when taking oral HRT containing estradiol (a type of oestrogen). We have a background risk of having clots due to estradiol in our bodies. Hence the increased risk of clots with the combined oral contraceptive pill as that also contains estradiol. However, taking transdermal oestrogen as a patch, gel or spray – when it's absorbed through the skin – does not increase your background risk of clots.

Heart disease, strokes & HRT

Transdermal, body-identical oestrogen, as opposed to oral synthetic oestrogen, does not increase cardiovascular risk. Micronized progesterones and dydrogesterone (which are both body-identical) also have a neutral effect on your cholesterol levels, your glucose metabolism and your blood vessel tone. This means, therefore, that your risk of strokes and heart disease is lower when taking body-identical HRT, compared with the synthetic versions. Anecdotally, global data is showing that, if HRT is started by those with a genetic predisposition to dementia (such as people who have the EP04 gene) in the perimenopausal years, that there is a correlation in dementia reduction. I am awaiting more peer-reviewed research regarding this, however.

It is important to note that if you have breast cancer or have had breast cancer, you can still have topical vaginal oestrogen HRT for vaginal dryness or genitourinary syndrome of menopause.

Endometrial cancer & HRT

The risk of endometrial cancer is greatly reduced in women who have a uterus when oestrogen is given in combination with progesterone. The progesterone can be supplied via oral capsules, a patch or a coil. If a woman has a uterus, and is using micronized progesterone administered vaginally (albeit off licence), it may actually improve endometrial protection. This is because it works at the uterus level and bypasses liver metabolism, therefore protecting against endometrial cancer when using oestrogen.

And, while we're on the subject of uteruses, a quick note about HRT and endometriosis: hormone replacement therapy can be taken by women with a history of endometriosis (this includes testosterone). However, individuals who've had a hysterectomy should be advised that oestrogen treatment can potentially reactivate some of their endometriosis symptoms. To combat this, they may be offered a little bit of progesterone or continuous HRT to help manage their symptoms. So, if you're an endometriosis sufferer who no longer has a uterus, please don't be deterred from taking HRT if you are experiencing menopausal symptoms; instead, chat through your options with your doctor.

Ovarian cancer & HRT

There is no increased risk of ovarian cancer in women with a uterus who take combined, systemic oestrogen and progesterone. Studies show that taking oestrogen on its own very slightly increases the risk of ovarian cancer, so oestrogen-only therapy is only given to women who've had a hysterectomy or have no uterus. If a woman has had her uterus removed but still has ovaries, she will also be given oestrogen-only therapy because a progesterone element to prevent thickening of the uterus is not needed. In this instance therefore, the small increased risk of ovarian cancer will remain.

Weight gain & HRT

There is a common misconception that HRT can cause weight gain but there is no data to show this to be the case. In fact, studies show that HRT helps you to manage a healthy weight because of improved energy levels and better sleep, which provides added motivation to exercise and follow a healthier diet.

HRT SUPPLY & SHORTAGES

The upsurge in demand for HRT is a beautiful thing, in my opinion – it signifies that more and more women are taking control of their own hormones – but in recent years it's led to serious shortages and supply issues, particularly with the newer body-identical products. This causes a great deal of worry and stress for all involved – thousands of women are reliant on oestrogen – it also prompts clinicians like myself to question whether the problem would be allowed to escalate if there was a country-wide shortage of insulin for those with type 1 diabetes or Viagra™. To me, it is yet another example of a patriarchal healthcare system effectively devaluing women's healthcare needs.

I've read a few articles effectively blaming the media for HRT supply issues, and maligning doctors for over-prescribing it. This is a ridiculous standpoint. We should be celebrating the fact that legions of women are benefiting from HRT, not bemoaning it. You'll certainly never catch me apologizing for signing off a stack of prescriptions for oestrogen and progesterone, that's for sure. Empowering a woman to make the right choices for her long-term health and wellbeing will always be my priority.

If you're faced with shortages and need to substitute your regular HRT, it's really important that you discuss this with your doctor. Absorption can vary between preparations, and there may be an element of trial and error before you find the level that works. This table provides a guide for oestrogen products, which most commonly see shortages, but the British Menopause Society (BMS) also advises on equivalent doses for progesterone, see the Resources section from page 217.

HRT oestrogen doses with equivalent progesterone doses

If you are taking systemic oestrogen as a patch, gel, spray or orally, this can be taken continuously (post-menopause) or sequentially (in perimenopause). If you have a womb, then the equivalent doses of progesterone listed below can reduce the risk of endometrial cancer and unscheduled bleeding.

PRESCRIBED OESTROGEN DOSE FOR ULTRA-LOW, LOW, STANDARD, MODERATE AND HIGH DOSE REGIMES

Application method	Ultra-low dose	Low dose	Standard dose	Moderate dose	High dose
Patch	Half a 25 microgram patch	25 micrograms	50 micrograms	75 micrograms	100 micrograms
Gel – pump	Half a pump	1 pump	2 pumps	3 pumps	4 pumps
Gel – sachet	Half a 0.5 milligram sachet	0.5 milligram sachet	1 milligram	1.5–2 milligrams	3 milligrams*
Spray	1 spray	2 sprays	3 sprays	4–5 sprays*	6 sprays*
Oral estradiol	0.5 milligram	1 milligram	3 milligrams	3 milligrams^	4 milligrams^

*Off-licence use

^Off-licence use

PROGESTOGEN DOSE PER LICENSED OESTROGEN DOSE IN THE BASELINE POPULATION							
Oestrogen dose	**Micronised Progesterone continuous sequential**		**Medroxy progesterone continuous sequential**		**Norethisterone continuous sequential**		**LNG-IUD (levonorgestrel intrauterine system) i.e. Mirena coil (52 milligrams)**
Ultra/Low	100 milligrams	200 milligrams	2.5 milligrams	10 milligrams	5 milligrams*	5 milligrams*	One – for up to 5 years of use
Standard	100 milligrams	200 milligrams	2.5–5 milligrams	10 milligrams	5 milligrams*	5 milligrams*	
Moderate	100 milligrams	200 milligrams	5 milligrams	10 milligrams	5 milligrams	5 milligrams	
High	200 milligrams	300 milligrams	10 milligrams^	20 milligrams^	5 milligrams	5 milligrams	

*1 milligram provides endometrial protection for ultra-low to standard dose oestrogen but the lowest stand-alone dose currently available in the UK is 5 milligrams (off-licence use of three noriday POP i.e. 105 milligrams, could be considered if 5 milligrams is not tolerated).
^There is limited evidence in relation to optimal MPA dose with high dose oestrogen; the advised dose is based on studies reporting 10 milligrams providing protection with up to moderate dose oestrogen.

OTHER PRESCRIBED TREATMENTS FOR MENOPAUSAL SYMPTOMS

Not all perimenopausal and post-menopausal people will pursue the HRT route. For some this is out of their control since they may suffer with medical conditions that prevent them from taking it. For others this is out of choice as they may simply want to try different options. The good news is that there are plenty of alternative treatments to consider, many of which are non-hormonal and can be prescribed by your doctor. I'm always happy to discuss all the whys and wherefores with my patients, and I'm sure your own doctor will be, too.

Gabapentin

This anticonvulsant medicine can help to combat hot flushes and night sweats. Its mechanism for alleviating these specific conditions is unknown, but we think it works on the hypothalamus, the section of the brain that regulates temperature. It does have side effects, though – especially if it's taken in higher doses – which include drowsiness, dizziness, weight gain and a dry mouth. It's a controlled drug that needs to be prescribed by your doctor, but please note that it may not be suitable for those who have stage three or four kidney disease, chronic obstructive pulmonary disease (COPD) or have an allergic reaction to gabapentin.

Pregabalin

This anticonvulsant and anti-anxiety medication can be prescribed, in low doses, to help with hot flushes. Side effects can include sleepiness, dizziness, headaches and blurred vision, and it's not recommended for patients who suffer with suicidal thoughts, COPD, chronic kidney disease or an existing addiction to pregabalin.

Clonidine

This non-hormonal drug is often used to treat high blood pressure (some brands are used for attention deficit hyperactivity disorder/ADHD) and is also licensed to help prevent hot flushes. Studies have shown that it is effective in this respect, but that it doesn't help with any other menopausal symptoms. One of its side effects is drowsiness, so it may well aid sleep and prevent insomnia. As it's an anti-hypertensive drug, I would not usually prescribe this to someone with low blood pressure.

Anti-depressants

Anti-depressant medications, such as selective serotonin reuptake inhibitors (SSRI) or serotonin-noradrenaline reuptake inhibitors (SNRI) are available on prescription and can really help with perimenopausal symptoms, primarily hot flushes. Side effects can include nausea, drowsiness, dizziness, headaches, blurred vision and low sex drive; doctors may not recommend SSRIs or SNRIs to anyone who has previously suffered side effects from them, or who is addicted to anti-depressants.

Menopause happens to women of all creeds, cultures and ethnicities!

MENOPAUSE IN BLACK, ASIAN & ETHNIC MINORITY COMMUNITIES

Menopause remains a taboo subject within ethnic minority communities which, by nature, tend to be very reserved and inhibited. I know from experience that many women in South Asian communities abide by a cultural attitude known as *purdah* – keeping things 'under the veil', in other words – which hinders discussion about gynaecological issues such as menstruation and menopause. These perfectly natural processes are deemed as dirty and unseemly – or are sometimes even sexualized – which leads to many women glossing over symptoms and suffering in silence, just to spare their blushes.

In addition, some of my patients regard the menopause as a Western phenomenon that only affects Caucasian women, and will often dismiss any tell-tale physical symptoms they experience themselves such as headaches, joint pain and vaginal atrophy. They may also gloss over emotional and psychological issues such as anxiety, paranoia, low mood or low self-esteem for fear of being seen as *pagal*, or mad. Others who are able to withstand sweltering temperatures in Delhi or Dubai will often play down vasomotor symptoms (related to blood vessel constriction) such as hot flushes or night sweats when they are back home in the UK, telling themselves they are mild in comparison and don't merit a doctor's appointment.

This whole mindset is really concerning because it means that women aren't benefiting from effective, life-changing treatment. When you hide things 'under the veil' you miss out on preventative healthcare, you're unable to benefit from treatment and, as a consequence, you can't pass on your knowledge and experience to others. People from South Asian, Middle Eastern and Black communities are particularly prone to type 2 diabetes, heart disease and osteoporosis as midlife approaches, and starting them on HRT before the age of 60 may actually reduce the risk of these complications, as well as improving their perimenopausal symptoms.

On average women of colour experience perimenopause earlier than their white counterparts and experience perimenopausal symptoms for longer

This situation can be exacerbated by the systematic discrimination that still exists within the healthcare sector, including a worrying lack of research relating to menopause and women of colour. However, while there's much work to do on these fronts, things are gradually improving. More Black and South Asian women than ever before are proudly telling me that they're receiving treatment for their menopausal symptoms, which makes my heart sing!

Menopause & Ramadan

Contrary to popular belief, Muslim women *can* continue to take all forms of HRT while fasting during the holy month of Ramadan. I've worked with the Royal College of Obstetricians and Gynaecologists, Muslim Women UK, and Imam Allama Arif Hussain Saydee MBE to produce guidelines for those who fast, but if you are concerned, you may also want to discuss things with your scholar.

The following types of HRT are not classed as having any nutritional qualities, so are perfectly permissible to use during Ramadan:

- **Transdermal oestrogen patches, gels and sprays** can be taken during Ramadan. The fact they're adhered or applied to your thigh or upper arm means that the hormones are absorbed through the skin, and head straight into your muscle and fat cells. You are not therefore breaking your fast. However, if you're using a gel or spray that needs to be applied manually on a daily basis, you may prefer to do this at the time of *sehri/suhoor* (before sunrise, so before you start fasting) or *iftar/iftari* (after sunset, when you break your fast).
- **Progesterone capsules** can be taken at *iftar*, once you've broken your fast. They should only be taken at night-time in any case, and they have the added benefit of helping you sleep.
- **A Mirena™ IUS coil** is inserted into the uterus so is not classed as nutritional, and does not break your fast.

- **Vaginal oestrogen** helps with genitourinary syndrome of the menopause (GSM), which can include conditions such as vaginal dryness and painful sex. Because it is applied topically – directly onto the affected area – it can be used during Ramadan and does not affect your fasting. Again, you may prefer to apply the cream or insert pessaries after *iftar*, following your evening prayers.

APPROACHING YOUR DOCTOR ABOUT MENOPAUSE

Women are far less likely to seek help with perimenopausal symptoms compared with other more obvious conditions, such as type 2 diabetes or heart disease. This is partly due to the fact that society still deems hot flushes, night sweats and irregular periods as 'women's problems' that are merely part and parcel of the menopause transition. This 'normalization' of symptoms, however, can make women feel obliged to soldier on without a firm diagnosis. If this is you, now is not the time to keep calm and carry on . . .it's time to go and see your lovely doctor!

That being said, I do appreciate that some people need to pluck up the courage to make that initial appointment – for many, menopause is a very sensitive and personal issue – so here's my step-by-step guide to putting those wheels in motion and getting yourself checked out.

Step 1: track your symptoms

If you think you may be perimenopausal (see pages 67–70), it's a really good idea to start tracking your symptoms. Try to do this for at least a month, up to a maximum of three months (by which time you'll have hopefully booked an appointment with your doctor).

By downloading a specialist menopause app (see Resources from page 217), you'll be able to track your symptoms and monitor any changes. From a clinical perspective, I really appreciate the fact that many menopause apps allow you to download your tracking data and take it along to your appointment. Analysing the timing, frequency and intensity of your symptoms can enable us to make a swift and accurate diagnosis.

If you're not app-minded, you can cross-reference your physical and psychological symptoms by reading this book, of course – head straight to pages 67–70 – or by accessing the NHS website. You can then jot down your observations in a diary, perhaps monitoring the timing and intensity of your hot flushes, or the regularity of your periods; anything, in fact, that you feel may be related to your fluctuating hormones.

All women in the UK are entitled to perimenopause/menopause care on the NHS and should NOT have to use private healthcare.

Step 2: prepare for your appointment

The more preparation you can do in advance, the better use you'll make of the time with your doctor. First and foremost, research your perimenopausal treatment options. If a patient arrives at my clinic with some basic knowledge of what's available to them, I might not need to start from scratch, and will therefore be able to spend more time discussing specifics and suitability.

You're essentially helping to direct your own consultation which, from my perspective, is always most welcome; it's a meeting of minds rather than a one-way process. You don't have to be a women's health expert, of course – leave that bit up to us! – but, as the old adage goes, information is power. By perusing this book, using an app, or browsing the NHS website, you'll be giving yourself a great head start.

From my experience, your first menopause-related appointment will involve general information gathering (you may not always receive hormonal or non-hormonal treatment at your initial consultation; this will often take place at the follow-up). Your doctor may also decide to check for any symptom overlap with other conditions, illnesses and deficiencies. Things like memory fog, hot flushes, anxiety attacks and low libido aren't always menopause-related, and can sometimes be attributed to other illnesses. Memory fog can be experienced by a patient with long Covid, for example, anxiety attacks can be caused by substance abuse, and hot flushes can sometimes indicate hyperthyroidism. As healthcare professionals, it's vital we think broadly.

Taking certain information to your appointment can be really helpful, too, not only to help us save time, but also to help us build a complete picture of you. You might consider gathering together the following:

- A list of symptoms (tracked via your menopause app, noted in your diary, or obtained from a Greene Climacteric Scale questionnaire, see Resources).

- Brief details of your immediate family's health history (such as diabetes, heart disease or cancer).
- A list of any prescribed or complementary medications you may be taking.
- Details of any allergies or intolerances you are prone to.
- A list of measures you are already trying (such as changing diet, stopping smoking).
- A blood pressure reading, if you have a monitor at home.
- Your latest height and weight measurements.

Some clinics will allow you to email the above information to your doctor in advance of your appointment; double-check this is the case by contacting the admin team or accessing the surgery's website. Mark your email for your doctor's attention, and it'll be forwarded to them prior to your consultation.

Step 3: find out what you're entitled to

It's your body, it's your menopause, so it's only right you take control! Make yourself aware of what care you're entitled to and, when you make your appointment, don't be afraid to state your preferences.

- You can ask to be seen by a doctor who specializes in women's/menopausal health (most surgeries have at least one nowadays) – this may mean a longer wait for an appointment, however.

- If you feel uncomfortable being seen by a male doctor, ask the receptionist for an appointment with a female doctor.
- Bring a friend or relative with you to your appointment or put in an advance request for the surgery to provide a chaperone; this can be another health professional.
- You can request a double appointment in advance for your first perimenopause-related consultation, but availability will depend on your individual surgery policies.
- You should have the option of a face-to-face, telephone or video consultation (although I'd recommend that your first perimenopause-related appointment is in-person).
- If English isn't your first language, ask the receptionist to book a translator for you or bring someone along to interpret for you.

Step 4: be proactive at your appointment!

As family doctors, we are committed to a person-centred approach, which means prioritizing the care and treatment that matters most to our patients, without judgement or assumption. For this reason, please don't be afraid to be upfront with your doctor when you see them; no one knows your body better than you, after all. The ideal appointment is a two-way process in which a doctor allows a patient to have their say, listens to their concerns and discusses options. Some diagnoses take longer to work out than others, but once you join up the dots and successfully prescribe the right treatment, both parties can experience a wonderful *eureka* moment.

It can be dispiriting for a patient to feel they're being fobbed off – I'm not a fan of that term, but I know it happens – or not taken seriously. Judging by some messages I receive on social media, this happens far too often. But rest assured, it is much less likely to happen if you follow steps 1, 2 and 3!

Asking your doctor the right questions can sometimes feel tricky, especially when appointment time is limited, but here are some common examples (all are subject to individual experiences, of course):

'I think I'm experiencing symptoms of perimenopause, such as . . . [then list your symptoms]. I've researched the hormonal and non-hormonal treatment options and would like your advice.'

'My quality of life has deteriorated since I've been having [then list your symptoms]. I've tried herbal treatments but they've not worked, so I'd like to find out more about HRT. Can you tell me about the risks and benefits?'

'I'd like to take oestrogen through the skin as a patch or a gel and, because I still have a uterus, I'd prefer to use body-identical progesterone.'

'I'm under 45 years old, so may I have an FSH (follicle stimulating hormone) blood test to exclude other causes for my symptoms?'

'I understand the FSH blood test might be repeated after six weeks, so I'll be around to have that done. I also understand that the FSH alone doesn't diagnose me as being in the perimenopausal phase; my symptoms (excluding other causes) can lead to the diagnosis . . .'

'I'm over 45 years old, I'm still having/not having periods, so I don't need an FSH (follicle stimulating hormone) blood test to diagnose that I'm perimenopausal.'

'I think my low mood may be due to hormone fluctuations. I'd prefer not to be prescribed anti-depressants and would like to discuss other options. I understand that HRT is a first-line treatment for menopausal symptoms, including psychological ones.'

MENOPAUSE IN TRANS & NON-BINARY PEOPLE

We need to be aware that research and conversations around menopause are usually framed around the experiences of cisgender women. For most individuals, this phase in life occurs in response to decreasing ovarian function; however, transgender and non-binary people can also experience symptoms of menopause even if the root causes differ.

AFAB (assigned female at birth) trans and non-binary people may take oestrogen blockers and testosterone in order to masculinize. Masculinizing hormone therapy does not usually cause menopausal symptoms but some individuals may experience hot flushes, night sweats, mood swings, lack of concentration, fatigue and sleepiness. Although masculinizing hormone therapy may decrease the risk of breast cancer, those who haven't had a complete subcutaneous mastectomy still need to remain breast-aware.

AMAB (assigned male at birth) trans and non-binary people may experience menopause-like symptoms (similar to those detailed above) if they are taking oestrogen-based hormonal treatment, which is often initiated before the age of 40.

Many of those in the trans and non-binary community receive little or no information about what to expect as they approach perimenopause and menopause. Moreover, there aren't enough fully trained specialists to help guide them through the process; as a consequence, a significant number of these patients do not get the care they need. Ideally, the management of their menopause symptoms – along with advice about NHS treatments available to them – should be overseen by a multidisciplinary team, which might incorporate the patient's doctor, a specialist in transgender health and a specialist in menopause care.

Positive steps are being taken to address this disparity, however, which I wholeheartedly welcome. In May 2022, the National Institute for Health and Care Excellence (NICE) announced plans to update its menopause guidance to include trans and non-binary individuals. This is encouraging news as it will undoubtedly benefit patients as well as professionals. For further guidance, see Resources from page 217.

Not all trans and non-binary people take hormones. A person can change their gender expression without any medical intervention.

BREAST CANCER

Breast cancer is very common and, in the UK, about one in seven women will be diagnosed with it in their lifetime. Early detection significantly improves the chance of successful treatment and recovery, which is why it is so important to examine your breast tissue on a regular basis (see pages 19–23).

Mammograms

Although younger women can get breast cancer, it affects more older people, and so anyone between the age of 50 and 71 who is registered with their doctor as a female and has breasts will be invited to have an NHS mammogram every three years. If you're 50 years old and have yet to be invited for a mammogram, it's perhaps worth speaking to your doctor. Another reason that mammograms are not routinely offered to younger women is that cancer cells appear white on a mammogram screening. Younger women have denser, oestrogen-rich breast cells, which also appear white on a mammogram. Therefore, it's harder to pick up white cancer cells on a white breast cell.

Self examination of the breasts is still of paramount importance!

A mammogram is an X-ray screening of breast tissue that looks for cancerous growths that are often too small to see or feel. The X-ray machine usually takes an image from above and an image from the side of each breast.

If thanks to genetic testing or knowledge of your family history you know that you have a BRCA1, BRCA2 or TP53 genetic fault, or Lynch Syndrome (a genetic predisposition to certain cancers), you can have an early breast screening. Your doctor can help you access the screening programme best suited to you.

Trans men and non-binary people will receive an invite for a mammogram if they have breast tissue due to either naturally occurring oestrogen, or oestrogen hormone replacement. A trans man who's had a double mastectomy and male chest reconstruction will not usually have a screening, but will still need to remain vigilant. Sometimes a small amount of breast tissue can be left behind after the operation, and it's always a good idea to keep an eye out for lumps or any changes to the skin.

Patients usually receive results from a mammogram after about two weeks, via a letter that will be copied to your healthcare provider.

Typical outcomes would be:

- All clear with advice to self-examine (see pages 19–23) and if you are over 50 years, to have another mammogram in 3 years.
- Unclear result with advice to have an ultrasound scan, an MRI and/or a fine-needle aspiration of a lump.

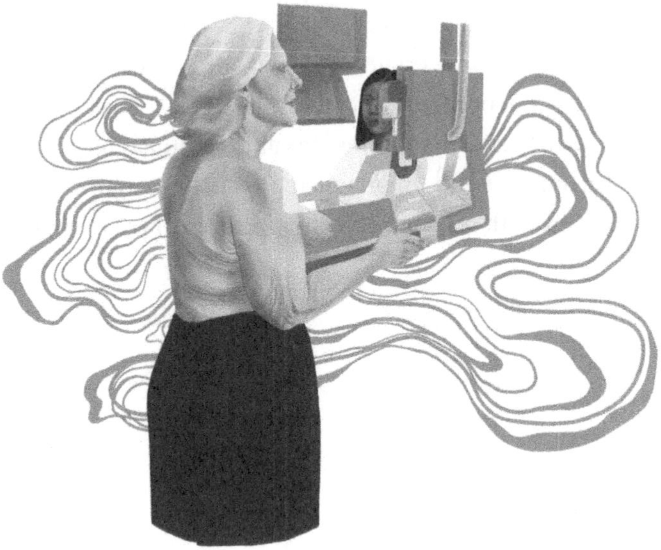

- Abnormal result with advice to see a breast cancer oncologist and a multidisciplinary team.

Anyone with an abnormal result will be referred for further tests and investigations (but this may not necessarily mean that cancer is present). Any treatment required will be handled by breast cancer specialists.

Post-breast cancer care

Post-cancer care for those who have suffered breast cancer will vary for each individual. You will receive practical and emotional support from your oncologist, but may also benefit from the fabulous guidance offered by Breast Cancer Now specialist nurses, Macmillan nurses and Cancer Research

UK (see Resources from page 217). They are so helpful and knowledgeable in all aspects of post-surgical care, and can offer advice about breast prostheses (artificial breast shapes), early menopause symptoms, sexual relationships, mental health support and financial/employment support. There is also a wealth of online information about breast health.

BREAST CANCER IN BLACK, ASIAN & ETHNIC MINORITY COMMUNITIES

Genetic differences and structural racism within many systems of healthcare, public services and public information sadly mean that breast cancer is significantly more prevalent in some ethnicities than in others.

Black women are disproportionately affected by breast cancer; compared with white women, they have a 70 per cent higher chance of developing the disease and are more likely to lose their lives to it. There is no conclusive data on breast cancer in other ethnic minority communities, but, knowing what we know about the ethnicity gap in other areas of health, I believe this just shows the need for more research to be done!

'Triple-negative' types of cancer, which tend to be more aggressive and harder to treat, are much more common among Black women. The reasons for this can include the following:

- Black women having denser breast tissue, so it is more difficult to pick up cell changes on a mammogram.
- Less awareness of breast cancer in the community.
- Late presentation and lack of understanding of screening in ethnic minority communities.

- High rates of inflammatory breast cancer, an aggressive disease in which cancer cells block lymph vessels in the skin and develop changes in their DNA, giving the appearance of a red, swollen or inflamed breast.
- High rates of obesity.
- Barriers to healthcare linked to geographical areas of deprivation.
- Racism in the healthcare system.

Spotting the signs and symptoms of breast cancer isn't always straightforward among Black women. Skin colour makes certain changes to the breast harder to detect – like redness and dimpling, for instance – so be particularly vigilant during self examinations (see pages 19–23). Medical professionals also need to be extremely aware of this when consulting Black, Asian and ethnic minority patients. Do flag this with your doctor if you feel concerned and please attend your mammograms when called for them.

Black women have a 70% higher chance of developing inflammatory breast cancer than white women

Whatever your race or ethnicity, please attend your breast cancer screening when you are invited at the age of 50.

DR NIGHAT'S TAKEAWAYS

1 Keep a menopause symptom diary, using an app or a notebook
It's so useful for both you and your doctor!

2 Never deny yourself treatment
There are risks and benefits to every medication and if you put up barriers, your health and wellbeing might suffer.

3 Don't suffer in silence
Visit your doctor and ask questions. If there's something you don't know, ASK. There's no such thing as a daft question!

4 Your lifestyle underpins all health conditions
Maintaining a good diet, taking exercise, reducing alcohol intake, stopping smoking and recreational drug use, relieving stress and investing in self-care is vitally important.

5 Share your experience
Share your experience within your community, your workplace, your family and your friendship group. Your lived experience increases awareness, drives change, prompts research, reduces stigma and fights taboos.

SHARING THE KNOWLEDGE

Throughout our lives we need to be able to keep checking and understanding our bodies. Know what is normal for you. Understand when something is not right and know when to go to your doctor to show your concern.

I want to emphasize that the stigma and taboo around women's health and women's biology ends with this book. Enough with the lack of diversity and inclusion in medical textbooks. Enough with misrepresentation of neurodiverse women and those who are differently abled. Enough of ignoring ethnic minority communities. Enough of undermining and gaslighting women's bodies and their symptoms. Enough with not providing adequate pain relief for smear tests, childbirth and hysteroscopies. Enough of not showing real-life body shapes. Enough of lack of data. Enough of medical misogyny, which is perpetrated by the patriarchy – including the patriarchy within us and our own misgivings about whether our pain is worth discussing.

Hopefully by now you've recognized that I have absolutely no qualms talking about breasts, vulvas, vaginas, anuses – the lot! I think it's so important for women to be queens of their bodies, and as queens we should be fixing each other's crowns along the way.

This book is not mine; it is my gift to you. Take the

knowledge within this book and share it like confetti with those around you.

Dr Nighat Arif

This book is my gift to you: take it, look after it, come back to it when you're ready, and know that you have the freedom to choose the care that suits you.

GLOSSARY OF WOMEN'S HEALTH

Abdomen The region of the body between the chest and the pelvis that contains the digestive and reproductive (or abdominal) organs, often referred to as the belly.

Abortion The termination of a pregnancy before term; this can be medically induced or spontaneous (known as miscarriage).

Adenoma A non-cancerous cyst or tumour resembling glandular tissue arising from the layer of cells inside organs (epithelium).

Adenomyosis A condition in which the cells that normally line the uterine walls (endometrium) develop in the muscular wall of the uterus tissue, but continue to thicken and shed as part of the menstrual cycle. Unlike endometriosis, these cells are always inside the uterus.

Amniotic fluid The clear, watery fluid that surrounds a foetus in the uterus, cushioning it as the mother moves around and allowing the foetus to move freely.

Amniotic sac The membranous 'bag' surrounding a foetus in the uterus, which is filled with amniotic fluid.

Anaemia A condition in which the concentration of the oxygen-carrying pigment (haemoglobin) in red blood cells is too low. It can result because there are insufficient red blood cells or because those that are circulating are defective. It is not a disease, but a feature of different disorders.

Anaesthetic Literally means loss of sensation. In medicine, anaesthetics are used to numb sensation in certain areas (local anaesthetic), or to induce sleep, for example for surgery (general anaesthetic).

Anal sex A form of sex in which a man's penis enters the anal passage of his partner.

Androgen Hormone that promotes the development and maintenance of male characteristics.

Antenatal Literally the time before birth of a baby. The term is mostly used to describe the care a mother receives during pregnancy prior to the birth.

Antibiotic drugs A group of drugs used to treat bacterial infections. They are sometimes offered to prevent infection if the immune system is impaired.

GLOSSARY OF WOMEN'S HEALTH

Bacteria (single = bacterium) Single-celled organisms abundant in air, soil and water, that are mostly harmless to humans. Some, such as gut bacteria, are beneficial and help break down food. A few, so-called pathogens, can cause disease.

Barrier method of contraception Forms of birth control, such as a condom or cap, that physically prevent a sperm reaching an egg.

Benign A growth or tumour that is not cancerous. It may continue to grow in situ, but it will not spread to other parts of the body.

Bilateral salpingo-oophorectomy Surgical procedure in which the ovaries and fallopian tubes are removed, often carried out as keyhole surgery.

Bi-manual examination A form of examination used to check internal organs in which the practitioner places one hand on the lower part of the person's abdomen and at the same time inserts two fingers into their vagina.

Biopsy A diagnostic test in which a small amount of tissue or a few cells are removed from the body for microscopic examination.

Birth control Any means of controlling fertility to prevent pregnancy, commonly described as contraception.

Bloating A feeling of fullness or swelling in the abdomen, possibly as a result of gas in the intestines, overeating, food intolerances or constipation.

Blood clot A mass of blood that forms if blood platelets, proteins and cells stick together. It can be carried around the body in the bloodstream or can become attached to the wall of a blood vessel (thrombus).

Body mass index (BMI) A means of assessing whether a person is a healthy weight by measuring both weight and height – weight in kg/lbs is divided by height in metres/inches squared – then plotting the calculation on a chart, which gives a number, for example anything between 18.5–24.9 is a healthy weight, above 25 is overweight and above 30 is obese.

Caesarean section/delivery Also called a C-section, this is an operation to deliver a baby through an incision in the abdomen. It is usually performed if a vaginal delivery is medically risky or because a birth becomes difficult (emergency Caesarean).

Cardiovascular disease Disorders and diseases that affect the heart and blood vessels.

Cervical mucus The slippery discharge secreted by the cervix that makes it easier for sperm to swim up the vagina; its consistency changes during the menstrual cycle.

Cervical screening A regular screening test offered every 3–5 years in women aged 25 –65 that assesses the health of the cervix. Cells are taken from the cervix to check for types of human papillomavirus (HPV) that can cause cancerous changes.

Cervix The opening in the lower end of the uterus that leads to the vagina.

Chaperone A person who accompanies another, for example to a medical appointment.

Cisgender (cis) A person whose gender identity is the same as that identified at birth.

Clitoris Part of the female genitalia, this is a small sensitive erectile organ located just below the pubic bone, partly enclosed by the labia.

Clot *see* blood clot

Coeliac disease A condition in which the small intestine is hypersensitive to gluten, the protein found in wheat, rye and barley. Eating gluten causes the immune system to attack and damage the gut tissues, and as a result the person cannot absorb nutrients.

Cognitive function Term used to describe mental processes involved with the acquisition of knowledge, information processing and reasoning.

Coil A small T-shaped device inserted in the uterus to prevent pregnancy. There are two types: a copper coil (intra-uterine device or IUD) and a hormone-releasing coil (intra-uterine system or IUS).

Combined oral contraceptive pill Contraception in the form of a pill that contains artificial versions of the naturally occurring hormones progesterone and oestrogen.

Conception The beginning of pregnancy marked by the fertilization of an egg (ovum) by a sperm.

Condom A sheath-shaped barrier device used to prevent pregnancy and prevent sexually transmitted infections. Condoms can be placed over the penis, or female versions (femidoms) are inserted into the vagina.

Contraception A means of controlling fertility to prevent pregnancy with barrier methods, coils or hormones.

Contraceptive injection An injection that releases the hormone progesterone into the bloodstream for longer-term pregnancy prevention; the effects can last between 8 and 13 weeks depending on the type.

Contraceptive implant Long-term form of contraception in which a small, flexible plastic rod is placed under the skin.

Contractions, uterine Rhythmic spasms of the muscles in the walls of the uterus that occur during childbirth.

Copper coil A small T-shaped implement inserted into the uterus as a form of contraception. This can be fitted at any point in the menstrual cycle.

Corpus luteum A cyst, or cluster of cells, which develops in the ovary during every menstrual cycle, just after an egg (ovum) leaves the ovary.

Crabs *see* Pubic lice

Cramps, period Known as dysmenorrhoea, cramps are painful sensations that can occur when the body releases the hormone-like substances called prostaglandins that cause the uterus to contract to expel its lining before and during a menstrual period.

Cyclical HRT A form of hormone replacement therapy (HRT) offered to women who have menopausal symptoms but who also still have their periods.

Depression A mood disorder that results in persistent feelings of sadness and hopelessness. Symptoms vary depending on the severity.

Diabetes A long-term metabolic disease characterized by high levels of blood sugar (glucose) in the body. Blood sugar is usually broken down by the hormone insulin. Diabetes can develop because the body produces no insulin (Type 1) or because the body cannot use the insulin it produces (Type 2) – the latter is often reversible.

Gestational diabetes A form of diabetes that can develop in pregnancy; this often resolves after pregnancy.

Diagnosis The process of identifying the nature of an illness by examination and assessment of the symptoms.

Diaphragm A barrier method of contraception that is fitted into the vagina to cover the cervix before vaginal sex.

Discharge Fluid that comes out of the body.

Early menopause This is the onset of menopause before the age of 40, and is also known as premature menopause or premature ovarian insufficiency (POI).

Egg A mature female reproductive cell (ovum) released from an ovary that, if fertilized, can develop into an embryo.

Ejaculation The action of ejecting semen from a male's body.

Embryo Human offspring in the process of development from fertilized egg to a foetus.

Emergency contraception This is contraception that can be given after unprotected sex to prevent a pregnancy. There are two forms: a person can take the morning-after pill, or a coil can be inserted.

Endometriosis A condition that occurs when microscopic cells similar to those found in the lining of the uterus – known as the endometrium – are distributed outside the uterus.

Endometrium The inner lining of the uterus.

Episiotomy A surgical cut that can be made at the entrance of the vagina to help a difficult birth and prevent perineum tearing.

Fallopian tube One of two tubes that extend from the top of the uterus towards the ovaries, in which fertilization takes place. The ovum moves along the tube towards the main body of the uterus and the sperm travels from the uterus towards the tube.

Family planning, *see* Contraception

Fasting cholesterol test A blood test to check for cholesterol levels, for which the person is normally asked not to eat for 12 hours beforehand.

Fertility A person or couple's ability to produce offspring, which is dependent on age and health.

Fertilization The point at which a sperm enters an egg (ovum).

Fibroid A benign, slow-growing tumour formed of smooth muscle and connective tissue that can develop in the uterus. There can be one or more and the size can vary.

Follicle A small cavity in the body, for example a hair follicle. In an ovary, follicles are small sac-like, fluid-filled pouches, each of which contains one ovum (egg).

GP A general practitioner, or family doctor, is a doctor who assesses and treats common medical conditions, and refers patients to other medical disciplines for more specialist treatment when necessary.

Gender The sex that a person identifies themselves as, such as male, female or non-binary.

Gender affirmation therapy Any of several therapies, psychological and physical, that are offered to a person to help them live in their preferred gender identity.

Gender diverse A place that accommodates people of different genders; also an umbrella term used to address the spectrum of different gender identities.

Genitals A person's external sex organs.

Gestation The period of time between conception and birth during which an infant develops in the uterus, normally 40 weeks or 9 months.

Gynaecological cancer A cancer that affects any part of the reproductive system of a female.

Gynaecologist Doctor or surgeon specializing in the branch of medicine that focuses on female health and the female reproductive system.

Hormone Chemical messengers released into the bloodstream by certain organs that have a specific effect on tissues somewhere else in the body.

Hot flush A common symptom of the menopause, caused by hormonal imbalances, in which a person experiences a sudden rise in body temperature especially in the upper body, often accompanied by sweating, and looks flushed.

Hyperthyroidism Also known as overactive thyroid, a condition that results in overproduction of thyroid hormones. Symptoms include increase in heart rate, appetite and sweating, as well as weight loss.

Hypothyroidism Also known as underactive thyroid, a condition that results in inadequate levels of thyroid hormones, causing tiredness, lethargy and weight gain.

Hysterectomy The surgical removal of the uterus. The most common type involves only the uterus and cervix; sometimes the ovaries and fallopian tubes are also removed.

Implantation The point at which a fertilized egg (ovum) attaches itself to the wall of the uterus – this normally happens six days after fertilization.

Incontinence The involuntary passing of urine, which can be caused by injury, weakness or disease of the urinary tract.

Infertility Inability to produce a baby. This can be a result of a problem in the male or female reproductive systems, or both.

Inflammation Pain, swelling, heat and redness in one or several areas of the body as a result of an injury or infection.

Insomnia The inability to fall asleep or to stay asleep for any length of time. Causes can be physical, psychological or environmental.

Insulin The hormone produced by the pancreas that controls blood sugar levels in the body.

Insulin resistance A condition in which the body's cells do not respond properly to insulin whether it's produced by the body, or injected (in those with diabetes).

Intercourse Also known as sexual intercourse, this is physical contact between two individuals that involves genitalia of at least one of them.

Intra-uterine device (IUD) Small 'T'-shaped, non-hormonal device (coil) that is inserted into the uterus as a form of contraception.

Intra-uterine system (IUS) Small 'T'-shaped, hormone-releasing device (coil) that is inserted into the uterus as a form of contraception.

Keloid scars A scar that continues growing after a wound is healed and can grow to bigger than the original wound.

LGBTQ+ Acronym used to refer to the group of people who identify as lesbian, gay, bisexual, transgender, queer or questioning. The '+' acknowledges that there are other sexual identities, such as intersex and asexual.

Labia majora The outer lips of the female external genitals.

Labia minora The inner lips of the female external genitals.

Labour The process by which an infant is born.

Laparoscopy A surgical procedure in which the interior of the abdomen is examined using a device called a laparoscope, which is inserted through a small hole ('key' hole) made in the abdominal wall.

Libido Level of sexual desire.

Lubricant An oily or slippery substance that can for example be used to reduce friction during intercourse.

MRI scan Short for magnetic resonance imaging, this is a diagnostic technique that produces cross-sectional or three-dimensional images of organs or body structures.

Mammogram A type of X-ray used specifically to examine the breasts for signs of cancer, offered as a form of screening.

Mastectomy Surgical removal of one or both breasts, usually to treat breast cancer.

Menopause The point in a woman's life when menstruation has ceased for 12 months, regardless of other symptoms.

Menstruation The periodic shedding of the lining of a woman's uterus that occurs if they are not pregnant.

Midwife A person trained to assist women in childbirth.

Migraine A type of headache characterized by recurrent attacks of severe pain, usually on one side of the head, which can cause a throbbing sensation.

Mini-pill Also known as the progesterone-only pill (POP), this is a contraceptive pill that contains only progesterone, which works by thickening the cervical mucus and preventing the sperm reaching the egg.

Miscarriage The loss of a foetus before week 24 of pregnancy.

Morning-after pill, *see* Emergency contraception

Multidisciplinary team Healthcare team that is comprised of a number of different specialties, who work together to assist with a person's medical care.

Myometrium The muscle tissue in the wall of the uterus.

Nausea Feeling sick or the need to vomit.

Needlestick injury Accidental puncture of the skin by a potentially contaminated hypodermic needle, which carries a risk of disease.

Neuropathic or neuropathy Disease or inflammation affecting the peripheral nerves, the nerves that connect to the central nervous system (brain and spinal cord).

NHS The UK's health system – the National Health Service – which includes all healthcare practitioners.

Non-binary A person who does not identify themselves as either male or female.

Obesity A state of being very overweight; a person with a BMI above 30 is described as obese.

Obstetrician A doctor or surgeon specializing in the branch of medicine concerned with childbirth.

Oestrogen(s) A group of hormones essential for the maintenance of female characteristics of the body.

Oestrogen-receptor-positive breast cancer (ER+) A type of breast cancer with cells that have receptors that allow them to use oestrogen hormones to grow – so a person can be given medication to reduce the hormone production as a form of treatment.

Off licence Use of a drug or other preparation in a way that is not typically recommended by the manufacturer, but that is still safe.

Oophorectomy Surgical procedure in which the ovaries are removed.

Oral medication Medicines or tablets that are taken by mouth.

Oral sex Sexual activity in which one person's genitals are stimulated by the mouth of another person.

Osteoporosis Loss of bone tissue that causes bones to become brittle/fragile so are more likely to fracture. This is a natural part of ageing, but women lose bone tissue faster after the menopause.

Ovarian cyst Abnormal, fluid-filled swelling that can develop on an ovary.

Ovary One of two glands, positioned either side of the uterus, in which eggs (ova) form and the female hormones oestrogen and progesterone are made.

Ovulation The process of the ovary releasing an egg (ovum).

Ovum (plural = ova) The mature female reproductive cell released from an ovary that, if fertilized, can develop into an embryo.

Patch An adhesive-plaster-like device that releases medication, for example for HRT or contraception, into the body through the skin; the patch is normally changed every 2–3 weeks.

Pelvis Large bony, basin-like frame at the base of the spine that surrounds and protects the reproductive organs.

Penetration Physical contact between two individuals in which a man puts his penis into the vagina or anus of their partner.

Penis The largest external male sex organ.

Perimenopause The time before the menopause when a woman has symptoms of the menopause, but is still menstruating; this can last up to a decade.

Perinatal phase The weeks immediately before and after the birth of a baby.

Perineum The part of the body between the entrance to the vagina (or the scrotum) and the anus.

Period Also known as menstruation, this is the periodic shedding of the lining of a woman's uterus that occurs if they are not pregnant.

Pessary Medical device placed into the vagina, to correct the position of the uterus or to deliver medication or contraception.

Physiotherapist Healthcare professional who provides physical therapy treatment to help prevent or reduce joint stiffness and aid movement.

Pituitary gland Situated under the brain, this is the most important gland of the endocrine (hormone-producing) system. Called the master gland, it controls and regulates all the other endocrine glands and many body processes.

Placenta The organ formed in the uterus during pregnancy that supports and nourishes the foetus.

Placental abruption Separation of the placenta from the wall of the uterus during pregnancy or labour before the baby is born; this is life-threatening to mother and baby.

Polyp A growth, often from a stalk, that projects from the wall of an organ, such as the cervix, uterus, or nose. Some are cancerous and need to be removed.

Polycystic ovary syndrome (PCOS) A condition that can cause cysts on the ovaries. Confusingly the syndrome can also cause other effects (such as excess hair, weight gain, oily skin, or irregular or absent periods) without the presence of cysts on the ovaries.

Post-menopause The life stage of a woman, or person assigned a woman at birth, after the menopause.

Post-natal The first weeks after the birth of a baby.

Post-partum The hours immediately after the birth of a baby.

Premature menopause Menopause that begins when a woman is under the age of 40 years.

Progesterone Hormone made in the ovaries that is essential to the functioning of the female reproductive system.

Progesterone-only pill (POP) *see* Mini pill

Progestogen drugs A group of drugs containing properties similar to naturally occurring hormone progesterone that are used in contraceptives.

Prolapse Displacement of an organ, for example the uterus, from its normal place in the body.

Puberty The time during which a girl (or boy) becomes sexually mature.

Pubic lice Tiny parasitic insects, often called crabs, that can attach themselves to the skin and hair of the areas around the genitals. Spread by close physical contact they cause intense itching; lice and/or eggs may be visible.

Pulmonary embolism Obstruction of one of the arterial blood vessels in the lungs by a blood clot. Clots can form in the lungs or be carried there from another part of the circulatory system by the blood.

Screening The regular testing of apparently healthy members of the population to check for signs of diseases.

Semen The sperm-containing fluid released from the penis during ejaculation/orgasm.

Sequential HRT A form of hormone replacement therapy for women who still menstruate that involves taking one hormone daily (oestrogen), then additional progesterone for part (normally half) of the month.

Sexuality A person's identity in relation to the genders they are attracted to, and/or how they identify their own sexuality. It also describes a person's attitude and behaviour towards sex and physical intimacy with others.

Sexually transmitted diseases (STDs) Diseases that are transmitted through sexual contact with another person.

Side effect The secondary response caused by a drug beyond the intended therapeutic effects.

Smear test Routine screening test offered every 3–5 years to all women (or those assigned female at birth) aged 25–65 in which cells are collected from the cervix to check for types of human papillomavirus (HPV) that can cause cancerous changes in the cervix.

Speculum Device placed in the vagina by a healthcare professional so that the cervix can be checked, and a smear test can be carried out.

Sperm The male sex cell that is responsible for fertilization of an egg (ovum).

Spotting Light traces of blood that can indicate the end of a period, or that are sometimes seen around ovulation.

Stress incontinence Involuntary loss of urine that occurs, for example, when a person coughs or lifts a heavy object, because the muscles at the exit to the urinary tract (sphincter) are weakened, for example after childbirth.

Surrogacy The process of carrying and giving birth to a baby for another person. The birth mother then hands over custody of the baby to that person.

Swab Small absorbent pad or cloth (generally sterile) used in surgery or by a healthcare professional to clean a wound, apply medication or take a specimen.

Synthetic A chemically made substance that imitates a naturally occurring product.

Systemic Medical treatment using substances/drugs that travel throughout the body.

Testosterone The hormone that stimulates the development of, and maintains, secondary male characteristics.

Tinnitus Continuous or intermittent ringing, buzzing or roaring sound in one, or more commonly both, ears.

Topical A medication or treatment applied directly to an area (of skin, for example).

Toxic shock syndrome A rare, but potentially life-threatening, condition caused by harmful bacteria getting into the body and releasing toxins. It is sometimes associated with tampon use in young women.

Trans man Person living as a man who was assigned female gender at birth.

Trans woman Person living as a woman who was assigned male gender at birth.

Transdermal Application of a drug through the skin, typically via an adhesive patch.

Transgender, or trans A person who is not living as the gender they were assigned at birth.

Transvaginal ultrasound scan An ultrasound scan carried out using a probe inserted into the vagina, *see also* Ultrasound scan

Trimester One of the three 'periods' of pregnancy, each covering around one-third of the pregnancy.

Triple-negative cancer An aggressive, fast-growing form of breast cancer in which the cells do not have hormone receptors that they need for growth.

Ultrasound scan A diagnostic tool that involves passing high-frequency sound waves through the body – the reflected echoes build a picture of the organs, or foetus for example, visible on a screen.

Unprotected sex Sexual intercourse with no form of contraception.

Urethra The opening, or sphincter, at the end of the ureter through which urine flows out of the body.

Urge incontinence The uncontrolled leakage of urine that occurs when a person feels a sudden urge to pee and is unable to stop the flow.

Uterine fibroids (leiomyomas) Noncancerous growths of the uterus.

Uterus Largest internal female reproductive organ in which a foetus remains during pregnancy.

Vaccine A medical preparation that is given to induce immunity to an infectious disease. Some require several doses to take effect and for others one dose provides life immunity.

Vagina The muscular tube, or canal, between the external female genitalia (vulva) and the internal organs of the cervix and the uterus.

Vaginal mucus Slimy substance secreted by the vagina that varies in consistency.

Vaginal atrophy Thinning of the vaginal walls, which can cause dryness and irritation.

Vaginal oestrogen A form of oestrogen (female hormone) that is administered in the form of a pessary or cream into the vagina.

Virus Simple, small microorganisms that replicate inside cells and can cause disease.

Vulva The external female genitals.

Vulvodynia Pain and discomfort in and around the vulval, vaginal and groin area. Can be generalised or provoked.

Withdrawal method A method to avoid pregnancy when the penis is removed from the vagina before orgasm/ejaculation to prevent sperm entering the vagina.

Womb The non-medical word used to describe the uterus.

X-ray A diagnostic tool that involves passing electromagnetic radiation of short wavelength and high energy through the body to view bones, organs and internal tissues.

RESOURCES

FAIR HEALTHCARE ACCESS FOR ALL

Women's health & disability

Sisters of Frida organization, a collective of disabled women: www.sisofrida.org

Trans patient training for doctors

GPs can access an excellent module on the Royal College of GP's LGBT Health Hub:www.elearning.rcgp.org.uk

The Gender GP online clinic also contains a wealth of useful information for physiciansand patients: www.gendergp.com

PHASE 3: YOUR MIDLIFE YEARS

Premature menopause

The Daisy Network offers advice and raises awareness of POI: www.daisynetwork.org

For a deeper dive into these conditions, I thoroughly recommend The Complete Guide to POI and Early Menopause by Dr Hannah Short and Mandy Leonhardt

Testosterone

To learn more about this hormone, watch Kate Muir's fantastic documentary Davina McCall: Sex, Mind & the Menopause (produced by Louise Perrie)

Menopause Mandate campaign group, working hard to effect change in the way testosterone can be prescribed: www.menopausemandate.com

Menopause Support: www.menopausesupport.co.uk

Skin-safe vaginal moisturizers & lubricants

Jo Divine: www.jodivine.com

Risks of HRT

National Institute for Health and Care Excellence, up-to-the-minute guidelines: www.nice.org.uk

Balance menopause app with Dr Louise Newson: www.balance-menopause.com/menopause-library/putting-the-risks-of-taking-hrt-into-perspective-with-sign-language

HRT oestrogen doses with equivalent progesterone doses

British Menopause Society, 'Management of unscheduled bleeding on hormone replacement therapy (HRT), p13 (table 2) and p16 (table 3), 2024: https://thebms.org.uk/publications/bms-guidelines/management-of-unscheduled-bleeding-on-hormone-replacement-therapy-hrt/.

This is a joint guideline prepared on behalf of the British Menopause Society, in partnership with the British Society of Gynaecological Endoscopy, British Gynaecological Cancer Society, Faculty of Sexual & Reproductive Healthcare, Getting It Right First Time (GIRFT), Royal College of General Practitioners and the Royal College of Obstetricians & Gynaecologists. And the BMS does hold the copyright for this document: Copyright © 2024 British Menopause Society. All rights reserved. Permission granted to reproduce for personal and educational use only. Commercial copying and distribution is prohibited.

Complementary therapies to control menopause symptoms

Complementary Medicine Association, a great information bank for patients and fellow GPs: www.the-cma.org.uk

Balance menopause app with Dr Louise Newson has a section on complementary therapies: www.balance-menopause.com

Acupuncture World Information Center, with accredited acupuncture therapists:www.acupuncture.org

The National Institute of Medical Herbalists, with a list of accredited practitioners: www.nimh.org.uk

Every Mind Matters initiative, with more information about cognitive behavioural therapy (CBT): www.nhs.uk/every-mind-matters

Women's Health Concern, offering a really useful CBT factsheet: www.womens-health-concern.org

Healthy eating

Dr Mary Claire Haver, a US-based obstetrics and gynaecology physician who specializes in women's nutrition: @thegalvestondiet on Instagram

Improving sleep

Sleepio, a handy sleep app: www.sleepio.com

Calm, another sleep app: www.calm.com

RESOURCES

Exercise

I often recommend the following exercise-related resources to my patients:

NHS Couch to 5K: www.nhs.uk/live-well/exercise/running-and-aerobic-exercises/get-running-with-couch-to-5k

Her Spirit: www.herspirit.co.uk

This Girl Can: www.thisgirlcan.co.uk

Perimenopause & metal health

Perimenopausal Depression: An Under-Recognised Entity by Jayashri Kulkarni: www.ncbi.nlm.nih.gov/pmc/articles/PMC6299176

NHS mental health advice; self-referral to NHS Talking Therapies services: www.nhs.uk/mental-health

Mind, a charity offering help with mental health issues: www.mind.org.uk

Menopause in trans & non-binary people

Rock My Menopause, an inclusive and informative resource offering guidance for trans and non-binary people: www.rockmymenopause.com

Gender GP (UK-based): www.gendergp.com

National Center for Transgender Equality (US-based): www.transequality.org

Tracking menopause symptoms

NHS symptom lists (search for 'perimenopause' or 'menopause'): www.nhs.uk

Health and Her, offering a menopause tracking app: www.healthandher.com

Stella menopause tracking app: www.onstella.com

Balance menopause app, my personal favourite, with Dr Louise Newson, a fantastic little tool that not only enables you to record and recognize your symptoms, but also allows you to interact with an online community of like-minded people: www.balance-menopause.com

Greene Climacteric Scale (GCS) questionnaire: this is widely available online, for example here: www.ardblair.scot.nhs.uk/your-record/electronic-reviews/menopause-symptom-scale-greene-climacteric/

Urinary incontinence & bladder health

Bladder Health UK, a charity offering some really helpful advice and information: www.bladderhealthuk.org

STATISTICS RESOURCES

Page 42: 8.9% of the residents of England and Wales did not have English as their main language in 2021 (Office for National Statistics 2021 Census,

29 November 2022. www.ons.gov.uk/peoplepopulationandcommunity/culturalidentity/language/bulletins/languageenglandandwales/census2021)

Page 70: 1 in 4 women said a lack of support for menopause symptoms in the workplace has left them unhappy in their job ('More than 1m UK women could quit their jobs through lack of menopause support' by Amelia Hill, the guardian website, 17 January 2022. https://www.theguardian.com/society/2022/jan/17/more-than-1m-uk-women-could-quit-their-jobs-through-lack-of-menopause-support)

Page 109: 81.9% of post-menopausal women have low levels of magnesium ('The Severity of Depressive Symptoms vs. Serum MG and Zn Levels in Postmenopausal Women', by M. Stanisławska, M. Szkup-Jabłonska, A. Jurczak, S. Wieder-Huszla, Samochowiec, Jasiewicz, I. Nocen, K. Augustyniuk, A. Brodowska, B. Karakiewicz, D. Chlubek and E. Grochans, Biological Trace Element Research 157, January 2014. https://doi.org/10.1007/s12011-013-9866-6)

Page 124: over 1/3 of women who visited their doctor with perimenopausal symptoms were offered antidepressants ('Menopausal women wrongly prescribed antidepressants which make their symptoms worse, warn experts' by Maya Oppenheim, the Independent website, 10 October 2019. https://www.independent.co.uk/news/health/menopause-antidepressants-symptoms-worse-hrt-shortage-a9148951.html)

Page 178: on average women of colour experience perimenopause earlier than their white counterparts and experience perimenopausal symptoms for a longer period ('What Experts Want Women of Color to Know about Menopause' by Beth Levine, Everyday Health website, 13 January 2022. https://www.everydayhealth.com/menopause/what-experts-want-bipoc-women-to-know-about-menopause/)

Page 196: Black women have a 70% higher chance of developing inflammatory breast cancer than white women ('New Research Highlights Disparity in Inflammatory Cancer Survival Rates', Rogel Cancer Center University of Michigan Health website, 10 December 2020. https://www.rogelcancercenter.org/news/archive/new-research-highlights-disparity-inflammatory-cancer-survival-rates)

INDEX

ACKNOWLEDGEMENTS

This book and my medical career so far would not have been possible without the help and support of so many people. It's true that it really does take a village! And in particular I'd like to thank the following people and organizations.

I want to say a huge thank you to my family. My parents, whose duas (prayers) and guidance continue to support me, and my siblings, Irfan, Imran, Saba and Ali, who will always be my best friends. My husband, Khalid, is a pillar of support, a dad to our three boys, and a soundboard for the choices I make. To my children, Haris, Qasim and Adam, who are my world and provide so much fun in my life. To the Pakistani women in my community: when I first arrived in the UK, they provided so much food, love, education and embraced us with open arms. These incredible women continue to teach me the facets of womanhood to this day.

When it comes to medicine and women's health, I am fully aware that I stand on the shoulders of giants, in particular Dr Louise Newson, who gave me the courage to push my understanding on HRT and menopause care and translate that to my South Asian community. Dr Annice Mukherjee made me understand the impact of hormones in women, and to Dr Radikha Vohra, Dr Aziza Sesey, Dr Liz O'Riordan, Dr Philippa Kaye, Dr Zoe Williams, Dr Larissa, Dr Sara Hyat, Dr Punam Krishan, Dr Naomi Potter – whose book with Davina McCall I contributed to – thank you for your support. Thank you also to my colleagues from the US from whom I learn so much: Dr Karen Tang, Dr Mary Claire Haver and Dr Rachel Rubin.

To all the people who have contributed towards getting this book into its current state, thank you. In particular, Dr Ajay Verma who has been immensely helpful in providing me with education and support when proofreading sections of the book, and Dr Kamilah Kamaruddin, who is a voice for trans rights in the medical community and gave her wise insight into the sections on healthcare for trans people.

A huge thank you to my family at Wellbeing of Women, especially Dame Lesley Regan, Janet Lindsay, who brought me on as an ambassador, and my fellow ambassador Rosie Nixon, for her constant support. Thanks also to Manjit Gill MBE from Binti Period, whose campaigning about periods is invaluable and who contributed her knowledge about the myths around menstrual cycles, and to Hibo Wardere and Nimko Ali OBE, whose advice helped me to write about FGM with clarity and authority. I'm eternally grateful for grassroots campaigners who do so much for women's health: Diane Danzebrink, founder of Menopause Support; Elizabeth Carr-Ellis From Pausitivity; and South Asian breast cancer campaigns and campaigners, Sakoon Through Cancer, Iyna Butt, Kreena Dhiman and Bep Dhaliwal. And thank you to the charities: The Eve Appeal, Jo's Cervical Cancer Trust, Breast Cancer Now, Lichen Sclerosus and Vulval Cancer UK Awareness who have been a wealth of information and have always supported my work.

Thanks to Jan Croxson, my agent, who found me in 2019, met me for 30 seconds and said she'd like to sign me. I was gobsmacked that somebody would take a punt on a hijab-wearing, slightly potty-mouthed, Muslim woman with three kids and take me into the world of media along with Borra Garson and Louise Leftwich. To Davina McCall for being so supportive and lifter of women.

To Kate Muir who originally asked me to be involved with *Davina McCall: Sex, Myths and the Menopause*. To Eleanor Mills who helped me to write about women's health and who brought me on as an ambassador for Noon.

A huge thank you to the BBC and ITV teams. Thanks also to my BBC Three Counties Radio team, especially Louise Parry, and Toby Friedner, who tried to teach me the art of presenting on a Sunday morning when I've had little to no breakfast and half a cup of tea, but with whom it's been an absolute blast to learn – there is more to presenting than I was ever aware of.

Thank you Baroness Sayeeda Warsi, Saira Khan, Anita Rani, Pippa Vosper, Lavina Mehta MBE, Meera Bhogal, Tessy Ojo CBE, for always championing my work. My HerSpirit friends: Mel Berry, Holly Woodford and Professor Greg Whyte, who literally motivate me to do exercise and get fitter, stronger, healthier in every way because I consume more chocolate than I should!

A huge thank you to my NHS surgery, in particular my supportive colleagues Dr Heather White, Dr Kirsten Riemer and Dr Lee Mitchell. To all my colleagues at OSD Healthcare who helped me set up a private women's health clinic to my own exacting specifications, even getting Entonox for pain relief in my coil insertion clinics. And to my NHS patients, who through their lived experience, have been more of an education than any medical textbook.

A massive thank you to Stephanie Jackson for believing in the vision of this book and taking on this huge gauntlet of a project. I'm so grateful to Jo Lake and Han, whose wisdom and advice I very much appreciated. I'm also grateful to Pauline Bache, Jaz Bahra, and Liliana Rasmussen for all their help, without Liliana's illustrations, this book would not have the soul that it does have.

My teachers at the Misbourne School, in particular my head teacher David Selman, who refused to make me head-girl so I could concentrate on my A-levels and become the first student from the school to go on to study medicine, thank you. Mrs Carol Taylor who provided me with mentorship and tissues as I cried in her office on a practically daily basis for fear of failure (she always had shortbread biscuits and tea); Ms Lorraine Cummings who helped me do my UCAS application to get into Queen Mary's University of London Barts and the London School of Medicine. And to all the professors, friends, lecturers at Barts who put me on my journey to becoming a doctor.

Finally to nine-year-old me, the little Nighat, who was so lost and had left everything she had known in Pakistan. She was in an alien world, never having the right clothing for the wet and cold weather, not understanding the new food and way of life, but she also gained all these freedoms and was able to not be hindered as a girl. Moving here, I felt a bittersweet loss of my life in Pakistan but I also realized a love of what I found in the UK. There's no other place like my hometown of Chesham. When I came here as that young girl I was constantly battling to try and find my identity, so I want to say thank you to that girl, because she persevered with a smile (still, when I'm nervous I smile, which is why I'm always smiling on TV!) and for gradually loosened the shackles of the patriarchy in a small way, being slightly rebellious and finding company in medicine. Because of that, this book is for all the other people who have a sense of loss of identity and loss of grounding – and who every now and then say to themselves, What am I doing? I hope that you can at least feel like you have a handle on and an understanding of your own body and how to best care for it, as a helping hand along the way.

ABOUT THE AUTHOR

Dr Nighat Arif is a GP specializing in women's health and family planning with over 16 years of experience in the NHS and private practice. She is based in Buckinghamshire, UK and is able to consult fluently with patients in Urdu and Punjabi. Dr Nighat is a medical educator and provides teaching to local trainee GPs as well as at national and international conferences. Dr Nighat was nominated for the National Bevan Prize for Health and Wellbeing to acknowledge her exceptional commitment to advancing wellbeing in her community. Dr Nighat has worked to raise awareness on menopause and women's healthcare in Black and Asian women; she presented her clinical work at the 'Menopause in the Workplace' Parliamentary committee hearing. She has also worked with Team Halo, a United Nations (UN) initiative to bring an end to the pandemic and presented at the G7 Global Vaccine Confidence Summit that led to her being awarded an Honorary Doctorate Degree in Science at London City University for Women's Health, Public Health and Inclusion. She is the honorary recipient of the 2023 SHE Award and received a Points of Light Award 2023 from the UK Prime Minister in recognition of her exceptional service to raising awareness for women's health in the UK.

Dr Nighat is the resident doctor on *BBC Breakfast*, ITV'S *This Morning* and BBC *LookEast*, and she hosts her own Sunday Breakfast show on BBC3 Counties

Radio. Dr Nighat was also a contributor on the Channel 4 documentary *Davina McCall: Sex, Lies and the Menopause* and has made guest appearances on numerous podcasts tackling taboos around women's health. Dr Nighat has regularly written for various publications including *Stylist*, *HELLO*, *Red*, *Good Housekeeping* and *Women in Medicine* and her work around menopause has featured in *British Vogue*. She is also an ambassador of the global charity Wellbeing of Women, Roald Dahl's Marvellous Children's Charity, The Good Grief Trust, HerSpirit, Sikh Forgiveness and Upon Noon. She lives in Buckinghamshire with her husband and three sons.

@DrNighatArif